WHEN YOU HOLD A PATIENT'S HAND...
DON'T WEAR A GLOVE

THE EXPERIENCES OF A MAINE RADIATION ONCOLOGIST

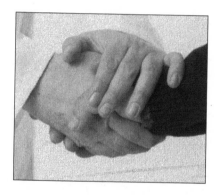

STUART GILBERT, M.D.

Thank you for what you do.

Stu Gilbert

STUGILBE@GMAIL.COM

TABLE OF CONTENTS

CARING FOR PATIENTS

DEDICATION

To my grandparents who made the courageous
decision to immigrate to the United States.

To my parents who through education and hard work
took advantage of the opportunities offered by our great
country and inspired me by their example.

To my wife Carol, my rock and the love of my life
who was always there for our growing family and
whose encouragement and invaluable assistance
made this book possible.

To my children, Scott and Alison and their spouses,
Lisa and Jeff, all of whom I am incredibly proud.

To my five grandchildren, Jesse, Hannah, Zach,
Megan and Noah for whom this book was written.

INTRODUCTION

I consider myself fortunate in so many ways. My parents provided me with the support and the opportunity I needed to help me strive for my potential. I was challenged throughout school and I learned not only from books but from their role modeling. I have also been blessed with a supportive and loving wife, terrific children, good health and a very fulfilling professional career as a radiation oncologist in Maine. Radiation oncology offered me an opportunity to treat patients and their families at a critical time in their lives when they are vulnerable and desperately in need of a helping hand.

Throughout my medical career I have had the privilege to meet some amazing and inspirational people who taught me a lot about life, how to live it and how to leave it. Sharing these experiences with family and friends brought me to the realization that we all learn something when we stand witness to the courage it takes to be a cancer patient and the physician who supports that journey. While writing these vignettes I noticed a theme; it is just as important, if not more important, to take care of the human being who is attached to the cancer as it is to treat the cancer itself. This led me to expand my collection of vignettes into this book about my experiences and life which I titled *When You Hold a Patient's Hand... Don't Wear a Glove.* I hope you enjoy reading it and benefit as much as I did from the wonderful people you'll meet.

In order to understand how I came to be the person and doctor that I am, I will tell you about my background and my parents, who helped shape my world. I will recount the journey of my father from life in Poland to him becoming a physician in New York. Then I will describe my upbringing in Brooklyn leading to my career as a radiation oncologist in Maine.

My Roots

"A PEOPLE WITHOUT THE KNOWLEDGE OF THEIR PAST HISTORY, ORIGIN AND CULTURE IS LIKE A TREE WITHOUT ROOTS." MARCUS GARVEY

I owe an incredible debt to my grandparents who made the courageous decision to leave Eastern Europe and start a new life in this great country. The members of our extended family, who did not emigrate, with very few exceptions, were murdered in the Holocaust.

My father was born in Bialystok, which is located near the Polish-Russian border. It had a vibrant Jewish population and was famous for the onion bagels that the Jewish bakers from the area created and named the 'bialy'. My father never spoke of his days in Poland but after he passed away I came across the book *Jewels and Ashes* written by Arnold Zable. It is about the author's parents who were both born in Bialystok and immigrated to Melbourne, Australia in 1936. Mr. Zable's father was born three weeks before my own father and his original family name was Zabludowsky, which was my paternal grandmother's maiden name. This book provided me with a literal picture of the village where my father was born and lived, and it was most likely told by someone who was a cousin to my Dad.

Zable told of the history of Jews in Bialystok starting in the 1700's, when Count Branicki, who owned much of the land in the Bialystok area, welcomed and protected the Jews so that they could build up the economy. Czarist Russia captured the area in the early 1800's and ruled over it for almost one hundred years. The Russians treated the Jews poorly and introduced anti-Semitic laws which restricted which jobs Jews could perform. Many were forced to resettle in certain sections of European Russia, called the Pale. Jews, in spite of being the majority of the population in Bialystok, could not vote in municipal elections, run for office or serve on juries. They were conscripted into the military at a higher rate than the gentiles and boys served from the age of twelve until they were twenty-five.

The Pogroms, which were organized and often officially encouraged, were rampages during which Jews were persecuted and massacred. Their goal was to 'encourage' the Jews to emigrate from Russia or convert. They began in earnest in 1881 and this started a mass emigration of Jews from Eastern Europe. Over the next forty years over two million Jews immigrated to the United States. The police and the army participated in a major Pogrom in Bialystok in 1906 in which seventy Jews were murdered and about ninety were seriously wounded. It was into this world that my father, the first of six children, was born to Chia and Lazar Gelbert, on December 29th, 1905.

Life was difficult under the Russians and did not improve in 1914 when the World War broke out and the Kaiser's German army captured Bialystok. During this time food and work were scarce but as Zable points out some of the German officers were Jewish so the Jews were treated fairly. In 1918 after the Poles kicked out the Germans, the Jews were once again mistreated. It briefly changed for the better in July of 1920 when the Bolshevik Red army captured the area. This reprieve was short lived however when one month later, the city was recaptured by the Poles and the Jews were harshly punished this time for supposedly collaborating with the Russian enemy.

My grandfather had had enough and made the momentous decision to leave for America with his fifteen year old son, my father. They left at the beginning of 1921 shortly after his sixth child, Frieda was born. My grandmother and the younger five children stayed with the Zabludowski family with the plan to bring the remainder of the family over in a few years. Lazar and Moishe Gelbert travelled to Danzig, now called Gdansk, where they boarded the ship SS Polonia and set sail on March tenth and landed in Boston on April tenth. Upon arrival, their name on the immigration papers was mistakenly typed 'Gilbert'. A few days later, when my grandfather noted the error, he contacted the authorities and they told him that he could legally change it back to Gelbert by going to court. The name remained

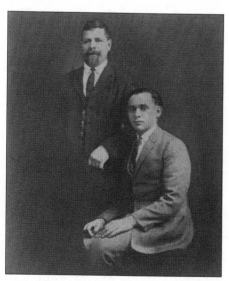

ABRAM LAZAR GELBERT AND MOISCHE GELBERT LISTED ON THE SHIP MANIFEST

MY GRANDFATHER LAZAR GILBERT
AND FATHER MORRIS

Gilbert. They were sponsored by a cousin, Ben Greenberg who owned the Hegeman Farm dairy in Brooklyn. They lived on the farm, earning their keep while Lazar also worked as a glazier to earn money to bring his family to this country.

My grandmother and the five younger children, ages seven to twenty, arrived in New York on the SS Arabic on March 16, 1927, after a six year separation. She went from Bialystok to Antwerp, probably by train and then boarded a ship, traveling in steerage for the long voyage to New York. Sea Sickness and often much worse abounded in quarters so close. When they arrived in New York they had to be examined to determine if they were healthy. If not, they could be quarantined or worse, be rejected and sent back to Europe. The ship line was required to give free passage to anyone and their family if they were too ill to enter the country. I have read about families who were faced with the awful realization that one of their children did not pass the health exam. Fortunately my family had no such difficulties. Today we feel sorry for a mother travelling alone with three young children as she boards a plane. I cannot imagine my grandmother's trip.

My father entered fourth grade at age fifteen and rapidly progressed in school as he mastered English. He went to high school at night and worked in the garment industry during the day at Simplex Cutting Machine Company, earning $75 per week, which was a great deal of money at that time. After high school graduation he went to Brooklyn Polytechnic Institute, a school for engineering. His plan was to study civil engineering but an instructor there told him that it would be very difficult for a Jewish boy in the 1920's to get a job in that field.

He decided to go to Marquette University, a Jesuit School in Milwaukee. I do not know why he chose this college perhaps because he had an Uncle Louis Zable, my grandmother's brother, who lived there. He completed four years of college in 1931 and then four more at Marquette's Medical School. During his eight years in Milwaukee he held down at least two and usually three jobs at a time, including waiting on tables for his meals, operating an elevator at night and working in a garage on the weekends. He also received financial assistance from his family and from Ben Greenberg. During his third year of medical school, the support from home dried up due to the Great Depression. He presented himself to the Jesuits to let them know that his circumstances had changed and he was unable to continue. In true Jesuit form, they responded by covering the tuition and allowing my father to pay it back over time. Not only was he able to finish and repay that gift but he made a generous annual donation for the remainder of his life.

He interned at St. Mary's Hospital in Grand Rapids, Michigan. During a Passover Seder many years later, Dad smilingly recalled that during Passover that year he went to the cafeteria for breakfast and the nuns behind the counter gave him a special plate with matzah on it along with eggs and bacon. He ate the eggs and the matzah and left the bacon. Following his internship year he returned to Brooklyn to open his family medical practice in 1936.

What happened to the Jews who stayed in Bialystok? In 1939 there were 60,000 Jews which was half of the total population. The Germans captured the city on June 27, 1941 and on the next day they locked one thousand Jewish men, women and children into the Great Synagogue and burned it to the ground. The German soldiers surrounded the building and shot any poor souls who tried to jump out of a window.

A few days later more than a thousand Jews from the educated classes were taken out of the city and executed. The remaining Jews were restricted to the Ghetto. In November of 1942, two hundred thousand Jews from the entire Bialystok region were concentrated into a camp outside Bialystok. From there they started shipping them out via railroad box cars to the Treblinka Death Camp. The Ghetto was emptied by February of 1943. At the end of the War, only nine hundred Jewish inhabitants of Bialystok had survived.

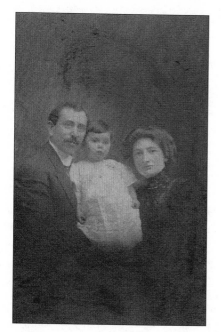

ESTHER AND AARON GISSIN
AND THEIR DAUGHTER SYLVIA

My maternal grandfather, Aaron Gissin, was born in Gomel, Russia, near Kiev. Sadly his older brother, like so many others was drafted into the army and killed in action. I never asked how it happened that he was able to avoid the draft. Members of the Gissin family had previously immigrated to Palestine where they founded the city Petach Tikvah, near Tel Aviv. In 1905, after a Pogrom in his town grandpa attempted to leave Russia to join them. He accompanied the wife of his cousin Boris Gissin who planned to reunite with her husband, but they were turned back at the Turkish border because of the Russo-Turkish War. Instead of going to Palestine my grandfather immigrated to the U.S. in 1906. He married my grandmother, Esther Terris in 1909 and soon after purchased a dental supply business in New York. My grandmother retired from the business at age 79 and my grandfather at age 85. They both commuted to work in Manhattan from their Brooklyn apartment each day on the subway. My grandfather was President of the Homler Society which was comprised of immigrants from Gomel who financed new arrivals from their hometown. I have fond memories of Shabbat dinner every Friday night at my grandparents' home where a typical meal consisted of gefilte fish or chicken fricassee, chicken soup with a matzah ball, boiled chicken and apple pie for dessert.

My mother, Sylvia Yvette Gissin was born on March 26, 1911 and was their only child. She graduated from New York University with a Bachelor's degree and then a Masters in History. She worked for her father's company as a bookkeeper since no other jobs were available during the depression. My parents met in 1936 and married the following year. My brother Warren was born in 1938 and I followed four years later.

My parents were true role models for their sons. My father was a General Practioner who cared for his patients and worked very long hours. He made house calls both day and night, delivered babies and treated patients even if they could not afford to pay. This served him well because after Medicare became law, in 1965, his income doubled. All of his elderly patients now became paying customers and they remembered who took care of them when they had no insurance. Many weekends my parents would be honored guests at a patient's wedding or bar mitzvah. He taught me a lot about caring for people. When I asked him if he felt sorry for himself seeing his first patients in the early morning and making house calls into the night,

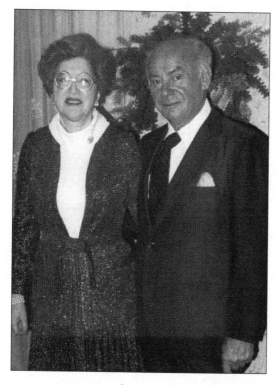

SYLVIA AND MORRIS GILBERT, 1977

he said that he felt sorry for the people who go to work and watch the clock so they could go home at five. He also said that he was getting paid for doing something that he would gladly do for free.

My mother was the backbone of our family and was committed to the community. She took care of my father's billing, answered his phone calls during office hours and made sure my brother and I studied hard. She was President of the local YMHA/YWHA, was on the local school board and was very active in several Jewish organizations.

My brother Warren was a hard act to follow. He was an excellent student and preceded me to Colgate and then to Tufts Medical School. He practiced urology in Brockton, Mass until his retirement in 2013.

My father died from colon cancer in 1979, nine years after his initial diagnosis. The tumor was small and his barium enema was initially read as normal. After I reviewed his x-ray and discussed it with my colleagues, it was determined that he needed further evaluation of an abnormality in his sigmoid colon. They found a small tumor that was completely removed with good margins so he did not receive adjuvant irradiation or chemotherapy at that time. Five years after the resection he developed a cough and a mass in his right lung was detected. Biopsy revealed a metastatic adeno-carcinoma compatible with the colon primary. He then received palliative radiotherapy and chemotherapy and enjoyed a good quality of life for four years until his death at the age of seventy-three. His impending demise gave us a chance to talk and reminisce and for him to give his final instructions to my brother and me. I asked him about his funeral and he stated that we should not feel sorry for him since he had a fulfilling life and he could not have asked for more. I then wrote and shared the following eulogy with him during our visit to Florida. He was pleased with it and encouraged me to deliver it which I did.

Morris Aaron Gilbert, M.D.
1905-1979

Don't shed your tears for me. Shed them for my cousins and fellow Jews who stayed in Poland and were slaugh-tered by the millions at the hands of the Nazi butchers.

Don't shed your tears for me. Shed them for the living who never achieved their true potential. Shed your tears for those of poor origins or who speak a foreign language and then throw up their hands and say "What's the use, I can't make it".

Don't shed your tears for me. Shed them for those who do obtain their educational and material goals, but don't know what to do with them. Shed your tears for those who forget their parents, who forget their families, and their Jewish Heritage. Shed your tears for those with the ability and knowledge to help but who don't.

Don't shed your tears for me. Shed them for those who are not blessed with a magnificent wife with whom to share a life full of love, achievement and fulfillment.

Don't shed your tears for me. Shed them for those who are not blessed with sons of the caliber of mine. No king or pharaoh ever left a greater legacy than my sons are for me. Shed your tears for those who are not blessed with the true love and respect from their sons, daughters-in-law and grandchildren.

Don't shed your tears for me. Shed them for those without a family such as the Gilberts. It can truly be said that this great country is a better place because Lazer and Ida Gilbert chose it for their new home.

Don't shed your tears for me. Shed them for those not blessed with dear and true friends with whom to share the happiness of life.

Don't shed your tears for me, but rejoice for me. Thank the good Lord above for the blessings he bestowed upon me of a long, fruitful, productive and satisfying life.

My Journey

"A LIFE IS NOT IMPORTANT EXCEPT IN THE
IMPACT IT HAS ON OTHER LIVES."
JACKIE ROBINSON

I was born on March 9, 1942, three months after Pearl Harbor and the entrance of the U.S. into World War II. Our family of four lived upstairs from my father's first floor medical office at 607 Pennsylvania Avenue in a then predominantly Jewish section of Brooklyn, called East New York. My childhood was a happy one in this lower middle class neighborhood.

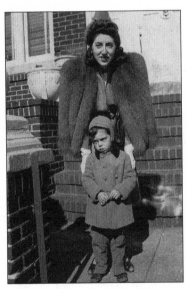
MY MOTHER AND ME IN FRONT OF OUR HOUSE

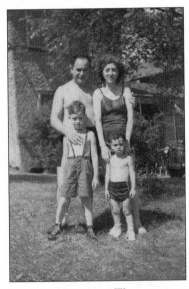
MY PARENTS, WARREN AND ME

I was an avid Brooklyn Dodger fan and knew all of the stats related to the team. That was the era when players usually stayed on the same team for their career. My favorite memory as a baseball fan was when the Dodgers beat the Yankees in the World Series in 1955 and was devastated when my much loved Brooklyn Dodgers moved to Los Angeles in 1958. I stopped following baseball at that time and only picked it up again years later when I moved to Boston and became a Red Sox fan.

In my youth I had the pleasure of following two greats of that era, Jackie Robinson and Sandy Koufax. Jackie Robinson joined the Dodgers in 1947 and was the first black major league player. He was thrilling to watch and the tension concerning his race intensified the excitement. He was very fast and often tried to stretch a hit and run for an extra base, but stealing bases must have given him a special joy, especially when he stole home. He played the mental game just as well when he distracted pitchers, already in motion, with a fake steal towards home from third base. In those days batters did not wear helmets and pitchers occasionally threw at him when he was in the batting box. As a second baseman, he experienced a few episodes when he was spiked or hit when a runner was trying to break up a double play or was trying to steal second. His first year was a tense and exhilarating one but also rewarding since at the end he was named 'Rookie of the Year'. Through my young boy's eyes it was incredible to see what this great man accomplished under unusual and challenging circumstances.

Sandy Koufax was another childhood hero. This Jewish boy from Brooklyn became the best pitcher of his era. A proud moment was when the Dodgers were in the World Series in 1965 and he chose not to pitch the first game because it was on Yom Kippur, the holiest day in the Jewish calendar. This was significant since whoever pitched on opening day could pitch the fourth and seventh games with three days rest in between. Don Drysdale pitched the first game for the Dodgers and gave up seven runs in the first three innings in a losing effort. Afterwards a reporter jokingly asked the manager if he wished that Drysdale was also Jewish that day. Sandy

Koufax lost the second game but won the fifth and, on only two days rest, won the seventh and deciding game, pitching two shutouts.

I did well in school and was placed in an accelerated program with sixty classmates who completed the three years of junior high school in two. At Jefferson High School I was on the tennis team and managed the football team. A memorable athletic event was at a tennis match with Boys High. My opponent was a fellow who had an amputation of his left arm just below the elbow. When he served he would put the ball inside his left elbow and throw the ball up in the air. It was hard for me to concentrate and to play aggressively against him. After I lost the first set my coach took me aside and said that our team had won two of the other single matches but lost a singles match and the doubles. My match would be the deciding one and he told me to stop feeling sorry for the other guy and to play more aggressively. I felt a lot of satisfaction when I went on to win my match.

Half of Jefferson High School's student body was black and most of the others were Jewish. One day I left the school through a side door. As I exited, the solid metal door accidently hit a black girl who was sitting on the outside step with her boyfriend. There were about twenty-five black kids standing around. She moaned that I hurt her and the other kids looked to her boyfriend to see what he was going to do about it. He started to come towards me in a threatening manner when Clint Weimer, the Captain of the football team stepped up and said that if the kid wanted to get me he would have to go through him first. Being involved with the football team certainly paid a large dividend that day.

I was sixteen years old when I entered my freshman year at Colgate University in upstate New York, near Syracuse. At that time it was a small, all male campus with an enrollment of three hundred and fifty in my class. I was young and immature and felt overwhelmed when I started college. Fortunately Colgate offered a close and intimate community with little place to hide. I made some lifelong friends, including my roommate Joe Simunovich and Jerry Northrup who helped me adjust and I thrived in my new community. I was an officer in our fraternity and managed the football team. My four years of college transformed me and gave me confidence.

In 1962 I entered Tufts Medical School in Boston. I worked hard and enjoyed the companionship of great classmates. I was the Editor of our Yearbook and Vice-President of our class. After graduation in June, 1966, many friends and classmates went off to other parts of the country for their internships. I began mine at Boston City Hospital, working every other night and weekend and was quite lonely until I met my future wife Carol Brecher that July. She was entering her senior year at B.U. and her dorm was a mile away from my apartment in Brighton. We spent an hour or two together on my way home most evenings. I asked her to marry me in November and we tied the knot eight months later on July 3, 1967.

During the spring of my internship year the house staff at Boston City conducted a 'Heal In' which protested the fact that we were paid only $3,600 a year, which was significantly lower than the other Boston hospitals. During the 'Heal In', all sick patients who presented to the Emergency Room were admitted for treatment and observation. I personally had twelve admissions the first day and with all the rooms full, we had patients lining the halls. We gave good care and admitted a lot of sick patients who would have routinely been sent home. The cost to the City was significant and they eventually increased our annual salary to $6,600.

I spent six years at Boston City Hospital, the first two on the Medical Service and the last four in Radiology and Radiotherapy. By the time I left BCH, I was boarded in both Diagnostic Radiology and Radiotherapy. In 1972 my young family relocated to Sheppard Air Force Base in Wichita Falls, Texas where I fulfilled my two year tour of duty as a Major in the Air Force Medical Corps. At that time all healthy men were eligible for the draft and I deferred my obligation until after I completed my training. The Vietnam War was still active and I was fortunate not to be separated from my family. This move to northern Texas was a real culture shock after living in the northeast for my entire life. After working long hours and nights in residency, I was able to enjoy spending time with my wife, three year old

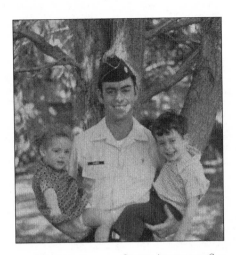

SCOTT, ALISON AND STU
AT SHEPPARD AIR FORCE BASE IN 1973

son and my one and a half year old daughter. We shared many happy hours getting to know this new area. In addition we were on a base with many young families in the same situation that we were in and we made several lifelong friendships.

My favorite 'war story' was when the Commander of the hospital wanted to crack down on the doctors for being 'shabby' officers. Many of us were moonlighting for the civilian hospital and specialty groups. The Colonel sent out a notice that no military physician could moonlight without his specific approval. The doctor who organized the coverage for the emergency room went to the civilian hospital's CEO and told him of the new situation. He said not to worry and went to his file cabinet and removed a letter. He gave him a copy of it and asked him to place it on the Commander's desk. The letter was from the Chief of Staff of the U.S. Air Force and addressed to Senator John Tower who was from Wichita Falls and then the Chairman of the Senate's Armed Services Committee. The General said that he was pleased with the mutually beneficial arrangement where the doctors of Sheppard AFB assisted the civilians of the city. He added that if anything should change this mutually beneficial arrangement he would like to be notified. Needless to say, the Hospital Commander did not follow through with his plan to stop our moonlighting.

The two years in the Air Force presented me with an opportunity to change my professional life in a very positive way. Here I was, fully trained and Board Certified, working in a busy regional hospital with two other radiologists reading x-rays. After a few months of sitting in front of my view box in my darkened office I became disenchanted with radiology because

I missed direct patient contact. I decided to go into radiotherapy and was offered a job in Wichita Falls. Instead of accepting, I applied to the Mass General Hospital in Boston for further training. Had I gone directly into private practice as a diagnostic radiologist from my residency at Boston City rather than go into the Air Force, I may not have changed my specialty to radiation oncology.

The world class Mass General Radiation Oncology Department was headed by the legendary Herman Suit and CC Wang. The staff and the fellow residents were terrific and I joined a group of Radiation Oncologists and Physicists who would remain my friends throughout my entire career. Dr. Suit was an exceptional clinician and researcher, produced extraordinary published work and enjoyed a worldwide recognition as one of the few greats in the field. During my training I attended the annual radiation oncology (ASTRO) meeting and was asked by Dr. Suit to join him for dinner.

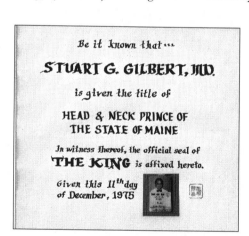

PLAQUE FROM CC WANG

I expected to see a big group in the lobby however when I came down to meet him it was only the two of us and we spent a memorably personal evening that I will never forget.

CC Wang was the chief of the clinical unit and I spent more time on his Head and Neck service than on any other. He was a great clinician, worked long hours and wrote many papers. I worked hard for him and took good care of his patients. I tolerated his quirks and we had mutual respect and admiration for one another. When I left Mass General I was really moved when he gave me a plaque that he personally created. It read that I was given the title of Head and Neck Prince for the State of Maine as declared by the King. He signed it with his Chinese seal, which he told me he had to dig out of storage.

During my second year at MGH, I was offered a position at the Maine Medical Center in Portland. I had previously attended a meeting at that facility and knew that it had a beautiful new department. Carol and I visited it and we jumped at the opportunity. Portland would prove to be a wonderful community in which to bring up our children and was only two hours away from family in the Boston area. Drs. Suit and Wang were disappointed that I was not going to continue in academia but I knew that this was the career opportunity that I wanted.

Maine Medical Center was an exciting place during the late 70's and early 80's. It was transitioning from a good regional hospital to an excellent medical center. During this time a large number of very well trained sub-specialists joined the staff and the drive to improve the quality of care was palpable. As an example, radiology added about two sub-specialists a year over a five to seven year period with specialties in angiography, nuclear medicine, neuroradiology, CT body imaging, bone, pediatric and chest radiography and so forth. These specialists did not add additional costs for our patients or the hospital and each built up their own new sub-specialty by giving talks and seeking out referring doctors in the hospital and the surrounding areas. Several other specialties had a physician who was the driving force in building an excellent department such as Carl Brinkman in Neurosurgery, Jean Labelle in Plastic Surgery, Ron Carroll in Medical Oncology and Peter Bates in Pulmonology to name just a few.

At MMC, we were fortunate to be the sole provider of radiation therapy (RT) services in Southern Maine. The RT facility at MMC was established through the vision, personality and hard drive of John Gibbons, the Chief of Radiology and my first boss in Maine. Rather than have two or three hospitals with Cobalt machines in Southern Maine that would divide up the patients, he convinced all seventeen hospitals in the area to agree not do RT in their facilities and to support one first class center at MMC. That center is known as the Southern Maine Radiation Therapy Institute, SMRTI. John Gibbons gave me very wise council when I arrived in 1976. He said, "You will remain a monopoly as long as you do not act like one".

I took the SMRTI agreement very seriously. When a radiology resident at the Osteopathic Hospital wanted to rotate through RT in the early 1980's I arranged it in spite of MMC not allowing osteopaths to practice in our hospital at that time. When challenged by the administration, I reminded them that the SMRTI was the radiotherapy department for all seventeen of its hospital members and that we had an obligation to be responsive to their needs, as well. Our Department also actively supported tumor conferences at other hospitals even when Maine Med's administration or the local medical oncology group expressed concerns. That policy has served the hospital well over the years by maintaining a strong referral base and the 'competing' medical oncologists at the Osteopathic Hospital and at Southern Maine Medical Center eventually joined the local Maine Center for Cancer Medicine group.

The State, to its credit, centralized RT in Maine to only five centers, Portland, Lewiston, Augusta-Waterville, Bangor and Presque Isle. This plan, written by a committee headed by my senior partner, Jake Hannemann, enabled RT to be within one hour of almost all Mainers and allowed the centers to have a large enough population base to justify first class machinery, radiation oncologists, physicists, dosimetrists and radiotherapists.

Our working relationship with the surgeons, medical oncologists and other specialists was exceptional. They were all willing and able to assist us with our medical and surgical problems and we went out of our way to respond to their needs. During those early years all the radiation oncologists were committed to building up our practice and our reputation in the community. Jake Hannemann, Chris Seitz, Jeff Young and I all served as President of the American Cancer Society's Cumberland Unit and gave frequent talks in schools and community meetings. Hugh Phelps served on the Freeport Town Council and was elected Mayor of Freeport. My fellow radiation oncologists and the Department's staff were superb and supportive of each other and it was a pleasure to come to work. If I had practiced in a suburb of a large city, no matter how good a radiation oncology department we had, it would always be considered a weak sister to the university centers.

We were the regional center and patients from Boston were often referred to us, as a respected first class Radiation Oncology Department.

An important measure of how well our Department did its job is how sat-isfied our patients and their families were with the care they received. In the mid 1980's, Bettsanne Holmes was the Chair of the Maine Med Board of Trustees. Her pet project was doing patient satisfaction surveys and us-ing them to improve patient care. During this time we had medical staff dinners and a lecture on the second Thursday of each month and over one hundred and fifty physicians attended. One month Mrs. Holmes present-ed the results of the patient survey and delivered it in a generic manner so that there was no mention of individual departments, inpatient floors or individual personnel. She reported that 91% of patients were pleased, while a few percent complained about the food, parking and noise in the hospital. At the end of her presentation, one of the general surgeons said that he thought this survey was not that useful since if a patient just deliv-ered a baby then she would be thrilled with the experience and everything would be wonderful. However, the feedback wouldn't be as positive if a patient had a serious medical issue. Mrs. Holmes answered that she too was concerned about how the reason for the admission could affect the pa-tient's response but was pleased to note that the department that had the highest patient satisfaction in the entire medical center was Radiotherapy. She added that these patients, with cancer, would have every right to be displeased.

Another experience occurred at Pen Bay Medical Center. At that time, I arranged to see a few follow-up patients from that area in the clinic after attending the monthly Tumor Conference. As I was examining a patient, she turned to a Pen Bay nurse in the room and told her that "The Radio-therapy Department in Portland is such a busy place but I always felt as if I was their only patient".

A year after I moved to Maine, Dr. Wang called to tell me that they had an opening on the staff at Mass General and asked if I would consider return-ing to Boston. I was honored by his offer but told him I loved both my job and living in Maine. Portland and then, Cape Elizabeth a year later, proved to be ideal places for us. We were warmly welcomed by the Jewish community, the medical community and our neighbors. I couldn't agree more with the sign at the State border, "Welcome to Maine: The Way Life Should Be".

Shortly after settling here, I decided to do a study on rectal cancer. I treated a couple of patients with very painful local recurrence from this disease and noted that they had a very slow, painful passing. Unlike tumor metastases to the liver and the lung, recurrent cancer in the pelvis does not lead to a quick demise and is manifested by invasion of nerves, the bladder and the bowel. The Gastrointestinal Tumor Study Group's paper was published at that time which showed that post-operative irradiation reduced local failure but did not increase survival when compared to surgery alone. At tumor boards I would recommend post-op radiotherapy but the surgeons would often respond that they removed the entire tumor and since radiotherapy did not increase survival then the associated morbidity of radiation therapy was not justified. I then decided to review all the cases of low rectal cancer treated with an abdomino-perineal resection (which involves removal of the rectum and anus and leaves a permanent colostomy) at Maine Med over a twelve year period and at Mercy Hospital over a fifteen year period. A total of 138 patients were analyzed. All had complete resection of the tumor, none had adjuvant irradiation or chemotherapy and none were lost to follow-up. If the tumor was limited to the wall of the rectum, only 20% recurred, however if the tumor penetrated the full thickness of the wall, then 50% of patients with negative nodes recurred in spite of total resection of the tumor. If the nodes were positive, the recurrence rate went up to 78%. The reason for this high failure rate of the tumor going through the full thickness of the rectal wall was that the distance from the outside of the rectal wall to the vagina and cervix in the female, and the prostate and bladder in the male was millimeters. Posteriorly, the rectum was millimeters from the pre-sacral blood vessels and nerves not giving the surgeon a lot of room to get clear radial margins around the tumor.

A total of 56 (41%) of the 138 patients failed and 57% of those who failed had only symptomatic local failure that lasted for an average of thirteen months before they died. Another 11% had symptomatic local failure for over a year and developed symptomatic distant failure during the last two months of their life. Thus, over two-thirds of those who failed had symptomatic local failure as the only or predominant factor and this lasted for over one year before their demise. Another 20% had only symptomatic distant failure and this led to death in a couple of months. Two-thirds of the local failures occurred within the first year following surgery while only one of the eleven symptomatic distant failures occurred during the first year after surgery. My conclusion was that even if adjuvant radiotherapy for rectal cancer did not increase the cure rate it is indicated for all lesions that extend through the full thickness of the rectal wall. This should avoid early, painful local failure that leads to a prolonged downhill course that averaged over a year. By avoiding or delaying local failure, we would prolong life and the mode of exodus would be much more humane since liver failure is generally painless. The novelty of my paper is that others reported the site of first tumor failure but did not document the duration and painful morbidity of local recurrence.

I first presented my paper at the Mass General the week before the national ASTRO meeting when all of the in-house presentations for the meeting were discussed. Dr. Suit was very impressed with my paper and the fact that I did it in private practice and was the sole author. It was well received at the ASTRO meeting and Dr. Suit invited me to present it at Oncology Grand Rounds at the MGH. He also invited me to moderate a GI scientific session at the annual ASTRO meeting when he was the President of AS-TRO. Another fortunate fact that prolonged my fifteen minutes of fame and established my reputation was that four of the leading GI radiation oncologists in the country were friends of mine at MGH. Lenny Gunderson became chief at the Mayo Clinic, Joel Tepper became chief at North Carolina, Tyvin Rich became the head of GI radiotherapy at the M.D. Anderson and eventually chief at the University of Virginia and Chris Willett stayed at the MGH for many years before becoming the chief at Duke. The four of them gave most of the GI refresher courses and wrote the GI chapters in the text books and all quoted my paper to justify the use of adjuvant irradiation following resection for rectal cancer that penetrated through the wall. Several years later physicians would stop me at regional and national meetings and ask me if I was the Gilbert who wrote that article and told me that they frequently quoted my paper at local tumor conferences. About five years after my paper was presented and published, the GI Tumor Study Group reported their randomized study of treating rectal cancer with surgery alone, or surgery with RT and/or chemo. The combination of RT and chemo not only had markedly reduced the local failure but also significantly improved survival. Thus adjuvant RT and chemo with surgery became the standard for treatment of rectal cancer that extended through the entire rectal wall. My paper was no longer needed to justify adjuvant RT.

Many years later I was informed how my paper influenced some of my colleagues. This incident involved the late Al Glickman, a prominent member of the local community who was born in Portland and had a successful career in Los Angeles. He returned to Maine where he continued his philanthropy, significantly enhancing the cultural and educational institutions in the area. His eighty year old mother developed breast cancer and had a lumpectomy in LA and the surgeon referred her to Dr. Chris Rose for radiation therapy. Dr. Rose recommended that she receive her thirty-three daily treatments at his office which was over an hour from where she lived. She asked if she could receive the treatments closer to her home and he said that the local radiotherapy centers did not have adequate quality control. Al then asked if she could receive the treatments in Portland and Dr. Rose asked who would give them. He replied that Stu Gilbert was at Maine Med and could take care of it. Chris Rose immediately responded that he knew me and that being treated in Portland would be fine. Of course Al told many people that this prominent Los Angeles radiation oncologist dismissed the other radiation oncologists in town but raved about me. My local reputation was definitely enhanced. A couple of years later I saw Chris Rose at an ASTRO meeting and thanked him for the referral. He trained at the Harvard Joint Center a couple of years after I was at the MGH and was unhappy with academia. After I published my paper, he and his fellow resident, Leslie Botnick, felt that I had shown that you can still go into private practice and earn the respect of the academic community. Chris Rose certainly did that, establishing a practice with Dr. Botnick in Los Angeles and eventually being elected President of ASTRO.

I was reluctant when Jake Hannemann asked me to take over his role as Chief of the Department in 1992. I declined at first because managing people or enforcing departmental or hospital rules made me uncomfortable. I preferred to lead by example and was disappointed when others did not step up to the plate. As I look back I realize that I took on more than was comfortable for me and should have delegated more administrative responsibility. All of my administrative meetings were from seven to eight A.M. and my meetings with architects and departmental meetings were usually from noon to one P.M. In addition, I was busy one evening a week with administrative meetings. All this time I maintained a full clinical schedule and the computer printouts showed that I billed more than any other radiation oncologist in the practice in spite of my many non-billable administrative hours.

At the time of my fortieth Medical School reunion we were asked of what professional achievement we were most proud. After much thought I wrote that it was the enlargement and development of the radiotherapy department during my tenure as chief. During my eight years the Bath facility came on line and our department was the driving force in getting the Scarborough campus started. We replaced all of our equipment and added two additional linacs, became fully staffed, especially in physics and dosimetry, and added an Impac radiotherapy computer system, steriotaxic radiotherapy, intra-cardiac brachytherapy, and prostate implants. Probably most importantly, we separated radiation oncology from radiology and hired our own Administrator. Our staff grew to seven radiation oncologists and our annual treatments went from 18,000 to 30,000 per year.

In 1998, after being chief for eight eventful years, I had what I'll refer to as my wake up call. At four P.M. a medical oncologist who had just admitted a patient with severe pain called me and asked me to see him. This was my third late afternoon referral in a two week period so I asked the medical oncologist how come he specifically asked to speak to me and not one of the other two doctors who were then in the department. He said he knew that if he told me he was concerned about the patient, I would willingly see him.

I felt very strongly that we should be responsive to the requests of our referring physicians. If they felt that a patient's pain was severe enough to warrant hospitalization for radiotherapy, then we should attend to him or her in an expeditious manner. I guess that was a lesson from my father's career where, after evening office hours he would go out to make house calls or occasionally get up in the middle of the night to see a patient in their home or meet them at the hospital.

When I evaluated a newly admitted patient at the end of the day I would briefly review the chart and available x-rays to determine how urgent the situation was and if the patient needed any additional studies before we could treat him. I told the patient and his family what to expect with radiotherapy and reassured him that his pain would be controlled in the hospital. By seeing the patient promptly, additional tests could be ordered on the day of admission and we can schedule our formal consultation and treatment planning either on the next day or after the test results are available. From the patient's point of view, when his family asks what was done in the hospital, he can say that he saw the radiation oncologist and he scheduled the treatment planning or ordered some necessary tests. The admitting medical oncologist has thus initiated the process and the patient and his family now looked to our department to arrange for the treatment.

Over the week following the medical oncologist's phone call, I did a lot of soul searching. I appreciated the fact that I had myself to blame for not delegating more to my colleagues. I realized that this old dog couldn't redesign himself and now that I had accomplished my major goals for the Department as far as administration, equipment and personnel, it was the right time to have a change in leadership. I decided to step down as chief and take over our satellite Bath facility which was serviced by one doctor. There I could run it as I saw fit.

The move to the Bath facility extended my professional life by several years. Here, the personnel acted like a family, looking out for and assisting each other without being asked, thus making it a pleasure to come to work each day. I developed a close working relationship with the referring doctors in the area by providing them with good prompt service. After a couple of years in Bath, one of my partners covered the Bath facility and later told me he had a very unusual day. He had two calls from referring physicians who asked for advice on how they should manage their patients and another call where the doctor was disappointed that the patient was not going to be seen promptly. I felt validated.

When I retired in 2008, three events were organized in my honor. The first was a surprise open house at Pen Bay Medical Center in Rockport. They had advertised it in the local newspaper and over one hundred former patients, family members of patients, doctors and hospital staff attended. I was given a Captain's chair from the hospital and other gifts, including one from the Tumor Board doctors and a painting done by the radiologist Peter Guistra. I was touched to receive many letters from former patients or their families who could not be there. A similar event was held for me in the Bath facility. My children and their spouses attended the dinner for our Department at the Woodlands Club and I was moved by the kind words that were expressed that evening.

The transition to retirement was a little more difficult than I anticipated. I set my retirement date three years in advance and I was dreading the thought since I loved my job; however, with six months to go I was ready. I retired on June 30, 2008 and really enjoyed the summer, playing a lot of golf and visiting family in Boston. In October my monthly radiotherapy journal came and I started to read an interesting article. After a few minutes I realized that that part of my life was over and I should move on. There were other things to read besides cancer. That thought was a little depressing since I had skills that were valued by society and that I loved to perform. I was not anxious to moonlight and cover other practices where I would not have any control over the quality of care provided. A couple of weeks later I ran into an old friend in Boston, Danny Dosoretz, who trained at Mass General a couple of years after me. He completed a paper on the MGH experience with testicular seminoma that I had started during my time at that hospital. He lived in Florida and built a company that owned about sixty radiotherapy facilities. His business model was to build a free standing high tech facility and place it in a suburb. He told me that he heard that I retired and said that he could use me. Many of his facilities were a one doctor office and he had to hire a locum to cover their vacations. Rather than get an unknown from a national agency, he would much prefer to have me. I told him of my hesitation to get involved with just any practice and he encouraged me to visit their Jacksonville office the next time I vacationed in Florida. I was surprised at how excited I was at the thought of working part time. I visited the facility and was extremely impressed with their radiation oncologist and her staff. I obtained a Florida license and covered there for several years. I also covered three Maine radiation oncology centers; Lewiston, Augusta and Presque Isle and really enjoyed the experience.

For the past five years I have had the perfect mix of part time work and free time to enjoy my family and to travel. After a year of doing locums coverage I asked a colleague when it would be time to fully retire. His answer was that I will know when the time comes. Early in 2013, I was writing a prescription for a drug I had prescribed for many years and as I was writing I was not sure if it was 20 or 25 mgs. I realized that it had been over a year since I last wrote a script for that drug. I knew it was time and made the decision to fully retire at the end of 2013.

Shortly after retiring from my full time career I realized that I was transitioning from a health care provider to a health care consumer. I had been relatively healthy other than for paroxysmal atrial fibrillation (A Fib), a condition that had been ongoing for about thirty years. I experienced two or three episodes a year, which were usually triggered by a second glass of wine or too much caffeine and it lasted for a couple of hours. An extra pill took care of the problem. My activity and the quality of my life were not affected until January of 2013, when my medications stopped working and I began to experience bouts of A Fib several times a week. My cardiologist tried a few different drugs but they did not control my rhythm so he recommended a cardiac ablation.

This procedure involves placing catheters in the groin and then cauterizing areas on the inner surface of both atria of the heart to destroy the aberrant nerves that are causing the arrhythmia. Cardiac ablation has only been around for about fifteen years with its technique evolving on a yearly basis just like computer or smart phone technology. It is effective in about 75% of patients and is very operator dependent. I was hesitant to undergo this invasive procedure being aware of the risks but the arrhythmias were preventing me from living an active life. My next decision was where to have the procedure; at Maine Med or at one of the major hospitals in Boston. I sought several opinions and decided to have it done in Portland by Dr. Andrew Corsello. My cardiac meds were discontinued forty-eight hours before my August 12th procedure and I entered the operating room in atrial flutter alternating with atrial fibrillation and a rapid ventricular rate. Four hours later I woke up in normal sinus rhythm. I am pleased to report that as a result of the ablation I have been free of any arrhythmias, am off of all my cardiac medications and I'm back to running two miles three times a week.

This experience, where I was confronted with the possibility of my active life coming to an end, was a very emotional one. The day after my procedure I read an article in the Portland Press Herald that Maine Med had to cut two hundred jobs in order to stem a negative cash flow. I knew how difficult that decision was for Rich Petersen, the President of Maine Med since he is a very caring person. I wrote him the following letter.

August 14, 2013

Dear Rich,

I read in yesterday's Press Herald that Maine Med had to cut a couple of hundred positions. These difficult but fiscally neces-

sary decisions enable the Medical Center to operate effectively and provide your excellent staff with the equipment and facilities to make miracles happen. I was a recipient of one of those miracles on Monday.

I have had paroxysmal atrial fibrillation since I came to Maine Med in 1976 but was able to control these episodes with medication. Thus the quality of my life was not affected until this January when my drugs were no longer effective. Despite trying other drugs my arrhythmia did not allow me to work out or do any aerobic exercise. On Monday, the 12th, Dr. Andrew Corsello did a cardiac ablation. I entered the OR with A. flutter, A. fib and a rapid ventricular rate and left four hours later in normal sinus rhythm. The quality of care and caring from Dr. Corsello and the staff in the OR and on R9 West could not have been better.

On difficult weeks like this, you must remember that your tough decisions allow these miracles to occur. Your efforts, with the help of Dr. Corsello and many others gave this 71 year old man a new lease on a full and active life, for which I am very grateful.

Keep up your good work and re-read this letter when you need to be reminded why you do this difficult job. My patient's letters got me through several tough periods during my oncologic career when I was painfully confronted with the limitation of what we can accomplish for some of our patients.

With respect, admiration and gratitude, I am,

Yours truly,

Stu

MY FAMILY

"THE GREATEST THING YOU'LL EVER LEARN IS JUST TO LOVE AND BE LOVED IN RETURN" NAT KING COLE

For me, that describes my family. I met Carol about one month after graduating from Tufts Medical School and in almost forty-seven years I have never doubted that she is my soul mate, the foundation of my adult life and my perfect partner. She taught third grade until she became pregnant with Scott. When Scott was sixteen months old, Alison was born. All through their growing up years she was an involved mother, assisting in their schools and volunteering in the community. For much of that time I was an absentee father during the work week. I was at the hospital from seven to six daily and attended two evening meetings a week, one for my administrative hospital duties and the other at Temple Beth El for ten years while I was on the Executive Committee leading up to becoming President.

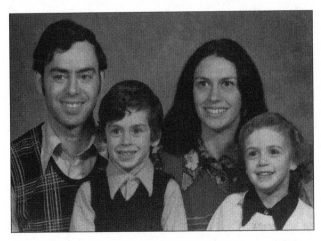

MY YOUNG FAMILY

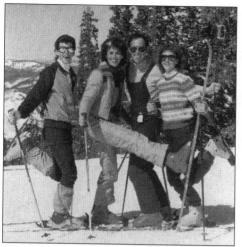

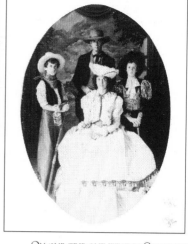

THE FOUR OF US AT VAIL   ON OUR TRIP OUT WEST IN COLORADO

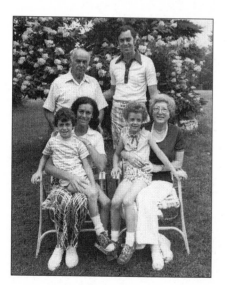

SYLVIA AND MORRIS GILBERT WITH CAROL, STU,
SCOTT AND ALISON AT CAMP KENNYBROOK

Family time for me came on week-ends, on our annual week long ski vacations out west, a visit to Florida to spend time with my parents, and our summer trips of one to three weeks exploring Canada and various parts of the U.S. Following these early summer trips, Scott and Alison went to Camp Kennybrook in Monticello, New York. My Dad was a part owner and the camp doctor which made it a really nice summer for all involved. My parents, my children and their cousins got to spend quality time with each other. Visiting Nana and Papa in their trailer may have been their favorite camp activity.

Every now and then a situation presents itself to remind us that priorities and allocation of time need to be re-thought. The following are a couple of personal examples. In our busy schedules, Carol and I felt it was important to have a Friday night Shabbat meal and evening together to anchor our family's values and heritage. One Friday I was at the hospital and was running late with sick patients. I was in my office after the last patient left and had a few dictations to complete before going home for the weekend. I called Carol at about 6:30 and told her I needed to complete the paper work before going home and she should feed the kids and I would be home in a couple of hours. Alison, who was about six at that time, had picked up an extension phone and said "but Daddy, it's Shabbat". I was stunned and realized that if it was my occasional Monday night tennis foursome, I would be on time no matter what. I realized that my family deserved no less. I told Carol that I would be home to join the family and then return over the weekend to complete my dictations.

In conversation you sometimes hear people describe the 'have to's' of their daily life. They have to mow the lawn, they have to pay bills or register their car. Family can never be a 'have to' it should happily be a 'want to'. I have to be the best physician that I am able to be, but I wanted to be the father that my wife and children deserved. My son Scott unknowingly gave me an opportunity, early on, to learn this important lesson. When he was in the eighth grade his State Cross country meet was scheduled for a Saturday up in Augusta, Maine. The Tuesday before, I was in the operating room lounge waiting for my radioactive implant to start. I told Dr. Annalise Andrews, an anesthesiologist, that some friends from New York were coming up to visit that weekend and that I wouldn't be able to go to Augusta to see my son run. It was a casual comment really, just sharing what the week ahead looked like. Annalise however, sat me down and educated me on the importance of being present in my children's life. Her lecture began by telling me that her youngest daughter was a track star in high school and was now a freshman in college. She reminded me that there is a small window in time to see your children compete in school athletic events and if you miss it you have blown it for your entire life. Fortunately my kids were just beginning their interscholastic sports and thereafter I made it a priority to attend as many of their events as possible, starting with the cross country meet the following Saturday. Cross country meets are not a great spectator sport until your child comes sprinting or dragging out of the woods but my friends from New York still enjoyed it.

Life is not a marathon but more like a relay race. You carry the baton for a short time and then pass it on to the next runner. I could not be more proud of Scott and Alison, my next generation. This circle of life gives meaning and immortality to our short stay on this planet.

Scott graduated from the Cape Elizabeth school system. In high school he earned twelve varsity letters as a long distance runner and was President of the student body. He went on to the University of Pennsylvania and then to Washington University Medical School in St. Louis. After this acceptance he decided that he wanted to delay his admission for a year to ski at Vail with his college roommates. I was apprehensive. When I was his age, if you took off a year between schools your Selective Service status changed from a student deferment (2S) to IA and you would probably be drafted and sent to Viet Nam. I feared he might enjoy the experience in Vail so much, that he would not return to medical school plus I didn't want a dependent for an extra year. I must say that my friends and relatives were supportive of Scott's decision. He assured me that he would not give up his Wash U spot and we agreed to let the Dean of Admissions decide. The Dean told him that he wished he had done that when he was young and granted the year deferral. During that year Scott crewed on a Windjammer in Camden during the summer, worked at Vail for the winter and backpacked by himself through Europe during the summer. To his credit he was able to support himself. His year off proved to be beneficial since during his four years at medical school he was more focused and involved than he had been in college.

I experienced a moment with both Scott and Alison when I realized they were not children anymore but very capable and respected adults. Scott's moment came for me at his medical school graduation. As President of his class he gave a speech that was remarkable and I was so proud to witness

39

the respect and admiration that the Dean, faculty and fellow students had for him.

A week after his graduation from medical school my son had his first lesson as a physician, and saw first-hand how important it is to be a caring doctor. My eighty-six year old mother had a diseased aortic valve that was causing intractable heart failure and the status quo was no longer acceptable. She agreed to undergo surgery but sadly did not do well post-operatively and wound up on a ventilator. The family took turns being with her. During Scott's three day vigil he called one night to say that the house officer was a complete jerk; "He came in, looked at the chart and monitors, then poked her as if she was a piece of meat and left." I told him to remember this experience and never forget that the patient you are treating is someone's loved one.

Another family experience that taught Scott an important lesson regarding how to treat a patient came when his Great Aunt needed to be hospitalized. Carol's father was the youngest of five children and the oldest were twin maiden aunts, Lottie and Mollie. Aunt Lottie died in her sixties from cancer and Aunt Mollie lived by herself in an apartment in Peabody. One day, when Carol visited her ninety-five year old aunt she found her sitting in a chair swollen from fluid retention. Carol said that she was not leaving her like this and wanted to take her to a hospital but Aunt Mollie refused. Carol asked Scott to come to her apartment to evaluate her since he was then a resident in medicine at the Beth Israel Deaconess Hospital. Scott visited and said that she had congestive heart failure and would be much more comfortable if she was treated with a diuretic in a hospital. Aunt Mollie said that she lived a good life and did not want to artificially prolong it. Scott promised her that she would not be put through unnecessary tests and procedures. She agreed to go and Scott put a note on the front of her chart to call him at any time concerning her care. Despite responding to diuretics, Scott received two or three calls a day from house staff who wanted to do more tests or interventions. He told of one call at two in the morning where the house officer wanted to transfer her to intensive care and Scott refused. The house officer challenged Scott asking how he knew what she wanted and Scott responded that the patient was very lucid and the doctor should ask her himself. Aunt Mollie responded to diuretics, was made more comfortable and ultimately transferred to a nursing facility where she was treated well by caring people. She died a few days later surrounded by her loving nieces and nephews. Physicians can make a huge contribution to how one lives and dies. By treating her with supportive care only, her doctors showed her respect and let her control the remainder of her life.

Today Scott is a nephrologist and is teaching at Tufts Medical School. He has been recognized as an outstanding educator by his fellow faculty members, the administration and most importantly by his students.

Our daughter Alison also had a positive public school experience at the Cape. She did well academically and athletically. She competed in track and held the all-time Cape records in the 100 meters, 200 meters, and the short and long relays. She was a tri-captain of the field hockey team and the starting forward on the basketball team that won the Maine Southern Conference championship during her junior and senior years.

Following graduation from Tufts University she served in the Peace Corps in Costa Rica for two years. We visited her two times in that beautiful country and during those visits I experienced the moment when Alison stopped being a child in my eyes and became a very well respected adult. We saw my little girl in the middle of rural Costa Rica with the closest English speaking person being thirty minutes away. Witnessing the love, affection and respect that Alison received from her community and visiting the pre-school program that she established was for me an eye-opening experience and earned her my greatest respect. Our concern for her safety in a foreign country was unfounded. I learned that the community took special responsibility for her well-being, making sure someone accompanied her home. I was told that if anything happened to her, it would be a serious black mark for the community. Her fluency in Spanish, even with a Costa Rican accent, has helped her get choice jobs over the years.

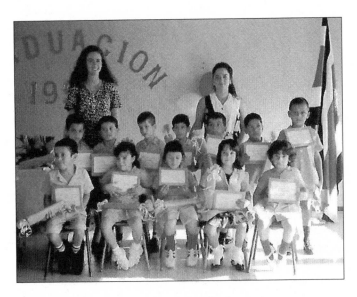

ALISON WITH THE
GRADUATING CLASS
FROM PRE-SCHOOL

Following her Peace Corps experience, Alison got a job working in the Head Start Program in Vail, Colorado where for two years she experienced a nice balance of work and play. A bonus was that she lived with her Cousin Adrienne which solidified a bond that was already strong. Then it was time to move on realizing that she needed some graduate degrees to get ahead. Over the next three years she earned two Masters Degrees in Social Work and Public Health at Boston University. Following graduation she specialized in domestic violence and worked for the District Attorney in Austin, Texas for a couple of years. When Scott and his wife, Lisa, announced her pregnancy with their first child, she wanted to come back East. She is now a domestic violence specialist working with the police departments in eleven communities in the western Boston suburbs. Carol and I take great pleasure in hearing about the respect and admiration that the Police Departments and the community have for her.

Both of our children chose truly exceptional spouses. Scott's wife, Lisa Weiner Gilbert is a gifted and very caring physician who now practices internal medicine in Lexington, Mass. They have three boys, Jesse (2002), Zach (2006) and Noah (2009).

Alison's husband is Jeff Tarmy, a wonderful man who works in business communications and spent five years working in China. I still get a kick out of seeing the expression on the waiter's face when Jeff orders in Mandarin at our local Chinese restaurant. They live in Newton Center in the house that Carol's grandmother bought and then sold to Carol's mother when Carol was six months old and then sold to Alison and Jeff in 2004. Alison's two girls, Hannah (2005) and Megan (2007) are the fifth generation to live in the house.

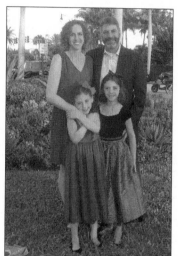

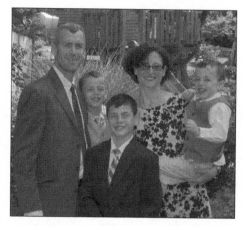

SCOTT, ZACH, JESSE, LISA AND NOAH

ALISON, JEFF, MEGAN AND HANNAH

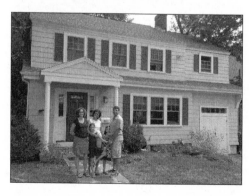

ALISON, HANNAH, CAROL, MEGAN AND JEFF IN FRONT OF THE FAMILY HOME

WHEN YOU HOLD A PATIENT'S HAND...
DON'T WEAR A GLOVE

**"BEFORE I CARE ABOUT HOW MUCH YOU KNOW,
I WANT TO KNOW HOW MUCH YOU CARE."**
JOHN C. MAXWELL

It is much easier to treat a cancer than it is to treat a patient and their family attached to that cancer. When confronted with the diagnosis of a malignancy and when their own mortality is at stake, patients realize that they have one good chance at addressing the tumor and they need to know that their physicians are good enough and care enough to give them their best shot for a cure.

I, like most physicians have never received formal training on how to 'care' for a patient. I was brought up to be a compassionate person, however, I have learned a great deal over the last thirty-five years from those very patients I was honored to have in my care. The vignettes that follow are a collection of my experiences with patients that have influenced me, taught me lessons which made me more sensitive to their needs and I believe have resulted in making me a better physician. I hope I will be able to convey some of these lessons learned to others.

Communicating With the Patient

"Tell me and I forget. Teach me and
I remember. Involve me and I learn."
Benjamin Franklin

Physicians spend many years studying the science of medicine but precious little time on how to talk to another human being who is emotionally as well as physically hurting and needs help and support. A cancer diagnosis intensifies the importance of that doctor-patient relationship. How a physician communicates with the patient is essential to providing the quality of care and caring that the patient deserves. There is an urgency to convey as much information as soon as possible but there is also the inability to digest it all at once. 'Cancer' is a word that paralyzes an otherwise thinking mind. Very often the initial physician, usually the surgeon, will start talking and the patient's mind will wander, thinking about how to break the news to their family and friends and what happened to acquaintances that had a similar diagnosis.

By the time the patient comes to the Radiotherapy Department they have dealt with the initial emotional trauma of their diagnosis and are better prepared to have an intellectual discussion regarding their management. In the past, since patients and their families often had little medical background, it was common for the doctor to tell them what the treatment would be. I believe that the best way to manage cancer is for the patient and their family to maintain control of their care with the guiding hand of the physician. The doctors may be the quarterbacks on the field but the patient should be the coach, who can send in plays and change the quarterbacks at any time. The doctor and nurse are there to explain what is going on in a manner the patient and their family can understand. This provides an opportunity for them to show respect and compassion for the patient while empowering him or her to take a more active role in their treatment.

In radiotherapy, we had the luxury of scheduling an hour and fifteen minutes for each new patient consultation. This allowed the physician ample time to have that all-important conversation because when dealing with cancer an extra effort has to be made to be sure the patient and family are fully informed. The more knowledgeable they are, the easier it is to manage their care. A recent article published online in the journal *Cancer* on March19, 2014 supports this approach. Dr. Neha Vapiwala, a radiation oncologist at the University of Pennsylvania did a study of 305 patients undergoing a course of radiotherapy treatments. One-third of the patients felt that they had active participation in the treatment decisions. Of these patients, 84% said they were satisfied with their treatment, 20% reported anxiety, 15% had depression and 33% had fatigue. In the two-thirds who did not feel they had any control or role in the treatment decisions, 71% were satisfied with their treatment, 44% reported anxiety and depression, and 68% felt fatigued. Dr. Kathryn Dusenbery, a radiation oncologist at the University of Minnesota made the following comment concerning the article. She said that "The main conclusion was that patients like to be part of the decision-making process. It is important for doctors to realize that we need to communicate with our patients and listen to them — we can't hear it too many times."

The patient who taught me the importance of first listening to the patient, understanding where they are coming from and what they need, and then tailoring my discussion for them was a forty-five year old school administrator. She was referred to me in 1989 by a general surgeon and had an early right sided breast cancer. He advised a mastectomy, but she refused and insisted on a lumpectomy. The surgeon and the patient agreed to have me see her and help with the decision. Mastectomy had been the standard of treatment at that time and lumpectomy and irradiation was just coming into acceptance. Definitive studies that demonstrated that they produced equal results had not yet been completed.

I saw her in consultation. She was very well informed of the studies on lumpectomy and irradiation. As we talked I learned that she had a very strong family history of breast cancer in that her mother and older sister both had had bilateral breast cancer in the pre-menopausal years. A third sister was younger than her and was well. Today we could use gene testing to determine if the family had a BRCA gene abnormality. During our one and a half hour discussion we talked about the high risk of developing another breast cancer after this one was controlled. At the end of our meeting she agreed to have a bilateral mastectomy and reconstruction.

Needless to say the surgeon was surprised. He put my letter recommending the bilateral mastectomies on the front of her hospital chart so that other doctors would not ask him why he was doing such aggressive surgery. After surgery the pathology revealed not only the expected tumor on the right but also a small, aggressive cancer on the left. I visited the patient in the hospital and she thanked me for my advice and added "Thank you for saving me from myself".

One year later I received a package in the mail. It contained a small silver bowl from this patient with a note:

Dear Dr. Gilbert,

Nearly a year has passed since I visited your office for a consultation prior to surgery for breast cancer. You probably do not remember me or my particular case because of the number of patients which pass through your doors. However, your meeting with me and your recommendation to me are landmark experiences in my life, as I'm sure they are to most patients who visit you.

Because of your meeting with me and because of your recommended course of action (bilateral mastectomy), I believe that I was given the optimum chance of long term recovery. Of course, one expects doctors to meet patients and ply their professional skill and knowledge. What was remarkable for me is the length and depth of discussion we had. As a result of the information you shared with me and the answers to my questions, I felt that I understood what had happened to me and what my actual circumstances were and needed to be. This probably seems the normal course of events to you, but my experience is that you are somewhat unique in your willingness to help the patient truly understand the disease and her particular situation.

Please accept this gift as a token of my deep appreciation for what you did for me and how you did it.

Sincerely,

I wrote the following letter back to her.

I have difficulty in expressing to you how deeply touched and moved I was by your beautiful and thoughtful letter and gift. I remember our discussion very well. During our meeting I noted that we were both educators, my role was in educating the patients so that they could understand their situation and make the appropriate decisions.

People often ask me how I can survive emotionally when I deal with patients with cancer day after day. My answer is that my profession provides me with an opportunity to assist people in a meaningful way at a very vulnerable and demanding moment in their lives. The gratification and fulfillment one derives is truly exhilarating but the frustration and disappointment occurs all too often. At these latter times, I save letters like yours so that I can re-read them. It is the best therapy to assist me in getting through those disappointing days.

I am glad to hear that you are doing well and I am sure that you will continue to do so. If I can be of any further assistance, please do not hesitate to contact me.

*Thank you again for your beautiful note and gift. The fact
that they came a year after our meeting, when the emotion of the
moment had past, made them mean that much more to me.*

Yours truly,

Stuart Gilbert, M.D.

I recently contacted this patient and she is cancer-free twenty-five years
later.

A more recent patient further illustrates the importance of communication.
In my semi-retirement I covered radiation oncology practices for friends
while they were on vacation. During one of these weeks I saw a sixty-two
year old man with lung cancer that had spread to a mediastinal node, to a
right rib and the right pelvic bone. He was seen in a lung cancer clinic and
a medical oncologist was scheduled to see him first. When he completed his
consultation, the medical oncologist told me that since the patient had metastatic disease he had scheduled him to start chemo the following week.
He added that radiotherapy (RT) could be put off for a while and so I did
not have to see the patient that day. I told him that I agreed with initiating
treatment with chemo but I would still like to see him and prepare him for
when he would need RT. When we met I sought out what he knew about
his tumor and his thoughts concerning his treatment. He said that he was
confused because his primary physician had referred him primarily for radiotherapy to the two painful areas, on the rib and pelvic bones, and assured
him that the local RT would relieve his pain. I initiated a discussion about
his disease and its management just as if I was speaking to a medical student. We reviewed his CT of the chest and the PET scan and I showed him
the normal anatomy and the cancer in the lung and the bones. We discussed
how the tumor spread from the lung to the bones via the blood vessels and
even though we could visualize only two spots on the bone, there could be
others that are too small to see. Then we discussed how the RT treats only

the area that it is aimed at and does not affect the rest of the body. Although RT is successful at palliating painful spots, the patient often returns weeks to a few months later with additional painful lesions that need treatment. Chemo however circulates via the blood stream and treats all parts of the body, those involved with the tumor, both grossly and microscopically, as well as those that are not. I discussed our coordinated plan. We would start with chemo and hope that he has a good tumor response. The quality and quantity of his life was most dependent on whether or not he had a good result from systemic therapy. If he tolerated the chemo well and the tumor responded both in the lung and the bones, he may not need RT to the bony lesions. However, if the bone pain persists then RT can be initiated at any time. By the completion of our discussion I believe the patient better understood his situation and now had the information that he needed to be able to have a major role in how his care would be managed.

EDUCATING THE PATIENT

Over the years I have developed a technique on how to explain complex concepts in a manner that is understandable to a patient and their family. The radiation oncologist has an advantage over his fellow colleagues since by the time we speak to the patient they have accepted their diagnosis of cancer and have already heard about lumps and lymph nodes from their other doctors. In addition, we have the advantage of knowing the pathology results and what exactly we are dealing with. The initial doctor's discussions involve dealing with the unknown, such as IF the nodes are positive, then we will do this and so on. Having the definitive pathology information allows us to tell the patient exactly what has to be done and why.

The following is an example of how I would inform a patient about her disease when her early breast cancer has been treated surgically with a lumpectomy and axillary (arm pit) node sampling.

The first thing I do is spend time to get to know her and her family. It is essential that the patient feels that I am treating her and not just the cancer.

This aspect of connecting on a personal basis with the patient is beautifully illustrated by a vignette in Dr. Rachel Naomi Remen's book, *Kitchen Table Wisdom*. She tells about a patient with cancer who spent many hours with his son hiking and climbing mountains. He told her that "In thinking back, I have a clear memory of many of these climbs, but no memory of anything my son said to me or I to him." She writes that "Many people live their lives in this way, sharing homes, jobs, and even families with others, but not connecting....Too often we even practice medicine this way. Side by side, patient and physician focus on the disease, the symptoms, the treatments, never seeing or knowing each other. The problem gets in the way and we are each alone." (*Kitchen Table Wisdom* by Rachel Naomi Remen, M.D., Riverhead Books, p.155-6.)

After taking a medical history and doing a physical exam, I meet with the patient and whoever accompanied her. I encourage her to interrupt me to ask questions and I suggest that her support person take notes. I start off my discussion by reassuring her that the surgeon removed all of the known cancer with the lumpectomy and that she may be cured with no further treatment. There is, however, a 20 to 25% chance that the tumor could return and it would be much easier and more effective to prevent recurrence at this point rather than to wait to see if there is clinical evidence of tumor failure. I divide up my talk into discussing the local recurrence issue and then the risks of distant spread of the tumor. I emphasize that radiotherapy only treats the local area and does not have any effect on cells outside of our focused beam.

The first question I address is "If the tumor was removed with clear margins why do I need any further treatment to the breast?" The answer is that in solid tissue a tumor grows circumferentially millimeter by millimeter by invading the surrounding territory. Clear margins on the skin or a solid organ like the liver will give us good control of the local tumor, however most breast cancer starts in the milk ducts and then invades through the wall of the duct into the surrounding tissue. Thus breast cancer cells can float some distance from where they originate via the ductal canals without any resistance and possibly set up new colonies in other areas. The breast acts more like a sponge rather than a solid piece of tissue. If the patient only had a lumpectomy, then 20% to 25% could have a local recurrence. These recurrences can be controlled with a mastectomy or a lumpectomy and radiotherapy in about two-thirds of the patients.

Then I discuss the risk of regional spread of the tumor. Most patients have probably heard a lot about lymph nodes but they usually do not know what they are. To best illustrate, I often use the following explanation. Nutrients and oxygen leave the small capillary vessels via the liquid portion of the blood, the plasma, and brings it to the cells. This tissue fluid in turn takes the garbage from the cells and returns it to the blood stream so that it can be removed from the body. Fortunately this fluid is not allowed to immediately re-enter the blood stream since it could be contaminated with infection, foreign bodies or tumor cells. The body collects this fluid in its own collecting vessels, called the lymphatics, which contain clear fluid and dumps that fluid back into the blood stream at the junction of the upper chest and lower neck region on each side. Before leaving the lymphatic system the fluid passes through several filters which hopefully eliminate any impurities that don't belong in the blood. If there is infection then these filters make antibodies to destroy it. An example of this action would be if one has a sore throat with the infected fluid draining toward the heart. If the filters function properly one would wind up with a sore throat and swollen glands (lymph nodes) and the infection would flow no further. If the infected fluid passes through these filters and dumps into the blood stream, then the patient can become septic with a high fever.

With breast cancer an important staging procedure is to evaluate the draining lymph nodes in the arm pit. If the nodes are positive for tumor deposits, then we know that the tumor has the ability to spread from one place to another via the lymphatics and this would have important implications on how to treat the malignancy. In some cases the pathologist will see individual tumor cells in the lymphatic vessels in or near the primary tumor or floating cells in the periphery of the nodes. In order for the patient to appreciate the significance of these findings I use the example of the allies invading Normandy. The cells in lymphatics in the breast are like men on ships on the English Channel. They have a means of transportation but have not shown their ability to invade. The cells floating in the periphery of the nodes are like a few soldiers landing on the beach, possibly an advance party, but they have not established a beachhead. When a sufficient force is established on the beachhead then they need supplies and reinforcements to maintain themselves. The tumor thus needs to attract a blood supply to nourish itself and grow. Studies have shown that 'floating cells' do not have a significant effect on prognosis while measurable tumor deposits, with a blood supply need more aggressive treatment.

The options for cancer treatment are surgery, radiotherapy, chemotherapy and hormonal therapy. It is important for all patients to have an understanding of what these modalities can and cannot do. Surgery is a local treatment that removes the tumor. All removed tissue is controlled and any tumor that is left is untreated and can recur. The surgeons are limited by what they can remove. For example, if the tumor goes around the spinal cord or another vital structure, then the tumor would be unresectable. If the tumor has already spread to a distant site then the surgery would be palliative and not curative. In breast cancer, surgery involves either removing the entire breast, which is a mastectomy, or removing just the lump with a margin. I tell my patients that every tumor is like the palm of my hand with fingers extending from it. The surgeon and the diagnostic radiologist cannot see or feel the extent of the fingers. Only the pathologist with a microscope can determine if the tumor reached the resected margin. After the pathology report is reviewed the patient may need a re-excision to achieve clear tumor margins. Some patients, especially those over the age of seventy may not need radiotherapy after an adequate lumpectomy.

Radiation Therapy is another local treatment. Only the tumor in the radiation beam is treated. Radiotherapy is able to deliver an intense dose since only a small portion of the body is exposed to the treatment beam. The advantage that radiotherapy has over surgery is that it can treat vital structures without removing them. For example, if the tumor involves the spinal cord, then the radiation oncologist can hopefully control the tumor with a dose of irradiation that can be tolerated by the adjacent spinal cord. For breast cancer, radiotherapy is given to most patients following a lumpectomy and to some patients who had a mastectomy. The RT is given either by external beam or by an implant. Radiotherapy for breast cancer is well tolerated since the tissue irradiated is the remaining breast tissue that protrudes from the chest wall and can be treated with tangential fields. With modern equipment and techniques we are able to deliver a full dose to the tissue at risk but avoid significant irritation to vital functioning organs such as the heart. The most frequent side effects are redness and irritation of the skin with occasional moist desquamation or denuded skin. Desquamation occurs when the skin is injured. A mild reaction is the pealing of the skin after sunburn. More intense injury can do damage deeper into the skin producing moist desquamation. This can be managed and should be self-limiting.

RT is delivered most commonly with five treatments a week for about four to six weeks. Each treatment is scheduled for a fifteen minute period with most of that time used to set up the patient on the machine. The actual radiotherapy takes a couple of minutes. The reason the treatments need to be fractionated over such a long time is that the radiotherapy irritates normal cells as well as tumor cells but normal cells can repair damage in a few hours while tumor cells recover at a much slower pace. I use the example of two twenty-five year old men. One runs five miles a day and is in great shape and the other is a couch potato. If you put them on a treadmill at one mile per hour (MPH) then they could both walk slowly without a problem, at thirty MPH they would both fly off but at five to seven MPH then the one who is in shape could stay on while the other would tire quickly and fall off. That is exactly what happens with radiotherapy and chemotherapy. Hopefully we treat long enough and hard enough to kill all the cancer cells but slow and easy enough to allow the normal cells to heal and survive. In other types of tumors such as those with bulky disease, we occasionally give chemo concomitantly with radiotherapy. Using the above example, the rationale of concomitant chemo is affecting the tumor more than the normal cells and thus makes the radiotherapy more effective. The chemo would be like putting football pads, a helmet, shoulder and hip pads, on the twenty-five year old who is in good shape but putting a twenty-five pound backpack on the couch potato. This added burden would enlarge the therapeutic ratio of damage to the tumor versus the normal tissue.

Chemotherapy is able to treat the entire body since the drugs circulate via the blood vessels. This provides us with a treatment that can not only treat the tumor that is evident but also the microscopic deposits throughout the body. With chemo we are limited by what the total body can tolerate. For breast cancer, chemo is given before irradiation since it treats the distant disease and will hold down the local disease. Since chemo gets to the tumor via the blood supply it is very effective for small tumors that metastasize via the bloodstream since those tumors are located close to the blood vessel wall where the chemo dose is the highest. In the area of the lumpectomy the blood supply is hampered by the post-surgical scar tissue. Consequently radiotherapy is much more effective at treating the local disease and the combination works well.

Breast and prostate cancers are amenable to treatment with hormones. The breast cancer cells that contain estrogen and/or progesterone receptors can be effectively treated with drugs that block estrogen. Tamoxifen can be given to pre- and post-menopausal women while the aromatase inhibitors, such as Arimidex and Femara, are only effective for post-menopausal patients. The duration of hormonal therapy is usually five years but can be longer.

I felt that the treatment planning process was another opportunity to educate the patient concerning his or her treatment. The Simulator is a CT scanner on which we place the patient in the position that they will be treated each day. At that time we manufacture cushions or masks to hold the patient in a reproducible position. We then take CT images through the area of interest followed by the physician outlining the tumor volume and the critical organs that should be spared on the simulator computer. The patient's initial response when they look at the images on the computer is that they do not know what they were looking at. Once I walk them through it and show them the CT images and point out the normal structures and the tumor and indicate how we plan to deliver the irradiation they become very interested and involved. Following the first treatment I would show them the final treatment plan that the dosimetrist and physicist produced. Showing the patient how we plan the treatments gives them a better understanding of the process. This enables them to appreciate the work and skills that our radiotherapists, dosimetrists and physicists bring to their care.

During my career I have witnessed a transition on how we use the surgical, radiotherapy and chemotherapy modalities. In the mid-twentieth century, surgery was used first. If the tumor was not completely removed or if the tumor recurred, then local irradiation was used. If the tumor spread to distant areas, then chemo was considered. Over the past several decades, physicians have been taught during their training what each modality can contribute and how the other specialties can make the treatment more effective if coordinated. The following examples illustrate this point.

Rectal cancer – The distance between the rectum and the vagina or prostate anteriorly and the pre-sacral area posteriorly, can be measured in millimeters. If the tumor has gone through the full thickness of the wall of the rectum and surgery alone is used then the risk for local recurrence is significant since the surgeon does not have a lot of room to get adequate margins. If adjuvant irradiation was given with surgery, then the local recurrence rate would diminish significantly since the radiation field would include a portion of the anterior structures and the pre-sacral nerves and vessels. We subsequently learned that the combination of chemo and irradiation produce even more effective results.

Acute lymphoblastic leukemia in children—Previously, chemotherapy alone was used to treat this disease and in the majority of patients the leukemia cells were cleared from the peripheral blood and bone marrow. Unfortunately, after chemotherapy was completed, almost all of the children recurred in the brain and spinal fluid. Physicians then realized that the chemo used at that time did not cross the blood brain barrier and the surviving leukemia cells could 'hide' from the chemo in the brain. A big breakthrough came when low dose irradiation was given to the brain after the patients were in apparent remission with clearance of leukemic cells from the blood and bone marrow. The result was a 50% cure rate. Today most low risk patients can be treated with special chemo drugs that do cross the blood brain barrier so radiotherapy is used mainly for high risk or persistent disease. Childhood acute lymphoblastic leukemia now has a cure rate of 80% to 90%.

To Tell or Not To Tell

"If you tell the truth, you don't have to remember anything."   Mark Twain

How much patients with cancer should be told about their disease has changed significantly over the past several decades. There was a time when the doctor would meet with the family to inform them of the diagnosis and not tell the patient. The word cancer was whispered to friends but was not discussed publicly. This was probably related to the belief that cancer was a death sentence and the medical community didn't have much to offer except supportive care.

Early in my career in Portland I learned how important it is for patients to be informed of their diagnosis. By fully understanding their situation, they are better prepared to make decisions regarding their care and how to live the remainder of their lives. They are also better able to tolerate the side effects of the treatments.

About thirty years ago I saw an eighty-four year old lady with a neglected breast cancer. The family had known about the tumor for some time but they and her doctor felt that she was too old for aggressive treatment. The tumor had now ulcerated through the skin and was getting infected. The physician, who referred her, stressed to me that the patient did not know she had cancer and it was important to the family that she not find out. Over the next two days I received phone calls from the patient's daughter, son, son-in-law and a brother, all telling me how important it was that mother not be told for fear that it would destroy her. Six family members accompanied her to the appointment. In the examining room I asked her what that was on her breast. She said that she had cancer and that it had been slowly growing for about two years. I told her that her family did not think that she knew and she looked at me in amazement and said "Do they think I'm stupid?" I had the nurse help her get dressed and arranged to have all the family members gather in our conference room. I told them that there was a terrible tragedy here. Mother has known she has had cancer for two years and has not said a word to anybody she loves about it. I then wheeled the patient into the conference room. I told them that we were dealing with a slowly growing breast cancer that showed no evidence of spreading to any other areas. Since this was before the modern era of hormonal therapy, I offered her a course of external beam radiotherapy. I told them that she would need to come in five days a week for about six weeks for her treatment. The patient quickly said that that would not be a problem; "John will bring me on Mondays, Sarah on Tuesdays" and so on. Needless to say the patient did not fall apart and the lines of communication were opened.

At the other end of the spectrum of life, is a young boy with an acute lymphoblastic leukemia (ALL). This was also about thirty years ago, before Maine Med had a first rate pediatric oncology service. He was admitted to the Dana Farber Cancer Center in Boston for treatment. While on the ward, another patient of similar age asked him what was wrong with him. He answered that he had a bad infection and was receiving antibiotics to get rid of it. The other child giggled and said that he must have cancer like him since he had lost his hair and was being treated at the Cancer Center. Later that day, the boy asked his parents if he had cancer and they admitted that indeed he did. He was so upset that he did not speak to them for several days.

I firmly believe in being completely honest and factual with patients but it is essential to present the information with sensitivity and to leave the door open for hope. After the extent of the tumor is discussed, I recommend a treatment plan and tell them what we hope to achieve as a result. When being bombarded with bad news the counterattack needs to begin. At this time I reassure the patient and their family that the medical team will not abandon them.

I made a special effort to have both the patient and their family in the room when I informed them of the tumor status. If I told the family in a separate room then they would not be certain what the patient knew and would have to think before they discussed the matter. To tell all involved at the same time keeps the lines of communication open and more supportive. As Mark Twain's quote stated at the beginning of this chapter, "If you tell the truth, you don't have to remember anything."

Listening to the patient and addressing their needs is important since they and their families are almost always overwhelmed at this point. The patient needs to be reassured that he or she is a normal person responding to an abnormal situation. Elisabeth Kubler-Ross wrote in her book *On Death and Dying*, that there are five stages patients go through when confronted with horrific news; denial, anger, depression, negotiation and acceptance. It is normal to go through these stages, sometimes more than once, but eventually we hope to get to 'acceptance' where we realize that this is the hand we are dealt and we are going to have to play it the best we can.

A Challenging Request

One of my most memorable patients was Angie Abraham, a seventeen year old high school student, who had a Ewing's sarcoma of the left femur. This tumor is an unusual lesion that is often found in the pelvic bones and the femurs. It occurs frequently in teenagers and young adults with a peak incidence between the ages of ten and twenty. She was a sweet, personable young woman and a great all-around athlete. The initial recommendation in Boston was to amputate her left leg and treat with chemotherapy. I evaluated her and obtained another opinion from Dr. Herman Suit, who was my chief at the Mass General and one of the world's experts on the radiation oncology of sarcomas. His recommendation was to treat with initial chemotherapy followed by concomitant radiotherapy and chemotherapy and amputate only if residual or local recurrent disease was detected. She was started on a course of treatments as recommended by Dr. Suit and while undergoing radiotherapy she set the Maine State girls high school record for the indoor shot put. My daughter, who was competing for Cape Elizabeth's track team at that time, commented to me that the she had the greatest hair, which was dark and curly. Little did she know that Angie was sporting a wig, and I saw no need to tell her.

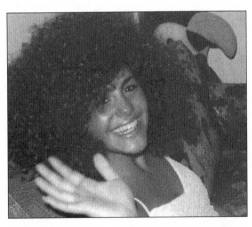

ANGIE ABRAHAM

Angie did well for several months with no recurrence or significant side effects. About six months later her mother, Sandy, walked over to our department while her daughter was getting a CT of the abdomen. She told me that her medical oncologist was concerned that the tumor had metastasized and then added that Angie wanted only me to tell her the results of the study. That was one of the most difficult requests of my career. An hour later I went over to radiology and found out that the tumor indeed had spread into the upper abdomen. I sat down with her and her mom and showed them the scans and quickly added how we planned to treat the spreading tumor. Through tears and hugs I answered each and every one of her questions.

She died about six months later but I was relieved that the tumor had not recurred in her primary site. Not amputating the leg certainly improved the quality of her life and her own body image. I would have been devastated if a local recurrence had led to her demise. Deering High School held an annual four mile race in her honor and a group of us from our department ran every year for the next few years. A scholarship fund in her name was established and students continue to benefit twenty-five years later.

I recently contacted Angie's mother and shared the above section with her. She responded with the following email on June 26, 2014.

> *Dear Stu,*
>
> *I read your email...and am still smiling. You have written this piece with love and deep understanding...thank you so very much. You have explained to me something that had bothered me all these years. I had always wondered what would have been if we had amputated her leg. Now I am very convinced that we did the correct action. I deeply thank you for this peace of mind I now have.*
>
> *Sandy*

I was disturbed that Angie's mother was bothered by the thought that not amputating her leg may have led to her demise. I believe the doctor's responsibility does not end with the patient's passing. Bringing closure and comfort to the family is important too. Although I have seen Sandy several times after Angie's passing her concern was never mentioned. For me, the reassurance that not amputating the leg did not affect the outcome came twenty-five years too late.

Angie's case is an example of a trend over the last thirty years to do less aggressive surgery and combine organ sparing surgery with radiation and chemotherapy. This has occurred as each specialty more fully appreciated what the other specialties can provide. The best example of this trend is the replacement of mastectomy with lumpectomy and post-operative radiotherapy. For some patients the limited surgery is not adequate to treat the tumor and more aggressive surgery is needed. For breast cancer, a lumpectomy is adequate for a lump but if there are multiple lumps throughout the breast, then the recommended treatment would be mastectomy.

The treatment of low rectal cancer, bladder cancer and cancer of the larynx present challenging situations since aggressive surgery requires a significant life style change often leading to a permanent colostomy, an ileal bladder (emptying into a urine bag on the anterior abdomen) or a laryngectomy with a stoma (hole in the neck). Amputations for tumors of the extremities also have a significant quality of life effect.

A good doctor-patient relationship is key to a difficult decision making process. When I would consult on a patient with a low rectal cancer I would review the findings with the patient and family members and then use an illustration that showed the location of both the tumor and the sphincter muscles that prevent incontinence. The patient is told that if the surgical resection does not remove all of the fingers of extension of the tumor, the risk of it recurring locally is significant. The other problem is that if the tumor is too close to the sphincter muscle, local resection could injure the muscle and this can lead to permanent fecal incontinence. I reassure the patient that we will try to avoid a permanent colostomy, if at all possible, but I did not want to 'kill him with kindness' by doing the wrong procedure. In order to try to save the functioning rectum I would recommend a course of radiotherapy and chemotherapy before surgery in an attempt to reduce the size of the tumor. The tumor should have significant regression from this upfront treatment and then the surgeon can reevaluate to see if a lesser procedure is possible. In about 20% of cases there will be a complete clearance of the visible and palpable tumor and the surgeon can then excise the local area where the tumor was and spare the functioning rectum. The patient however needs to be aware that we will do whatever we can to minimize the extent of the surgery without compromising the chances for eradicating the tumor. I have found that if the patients are convinced that the physicians really tried to save the functioning rectum and they were involved in the decision process, they would more readily accept the recommendation of a permanent colostomy. Whenever an organ sparing surgery is performed, the patient needs to be carefully followed to detect any recurrence and then treat it promptly. All physicians dread the possibility of having a patient fail due to incomplete treatment. Those cases have been a rarity in my career but the possibility keeps one up at night.

I have often been asked how I can deal with only patients who have cancer. "Isn't it depressing?" My response is that 50% of my patients will be cured and there is no greater feeling than guiding a patient successfully through the nightmare of cancer. Those who have widespread disease present a different scenario. It is like a relief pitcher in baseball coming into the game in the seventh inning with his team losing 7-0. If he can pitch two good innings then we know he did all he could do. I derived a great deal of satisfaction at prolonging a patient's life and providing him a pain free, dignified end of life.

I was mentally prepared for recurrences in patients who had a poor prognosis such as those with advanced lung cancer, pancreatic or other such tumors. It was when a patient with a favorable prognosis recurred that I had a more difficult time. When asked which patients affected me the most, I said children with cancer and young adults who had an avoidable smoking related malignancy. In the early 1980's I treated three patients who were in the prime of their lives. They all had malignant brain tumors that were difficult to control. One patient was the general manager of a large factory, another was a school teacher and the third was a concert pianist. The latter asked me if she could still perform after her surgery and radiotherapy. I told her that would be the ultimate neurological test but I was hopeful that she could. We were using a new protocol for brain tumors at that time which consisted of combined RT with chemo. All three patients tolerated their treatments well and returned to work. At one year they were all doing well and there was no evidence of tumor growth on the scans. I was optimistic that the new protocol may be a major advance in treating this disease. Over the next six months, all three recurred and I was devastated. Today we treat many brain tumors with combined radiotherapy and chemo but these tumors are still very difficult to control.

Friends and patients occasionally remarked that after being in the oncology field for so many years, dealing with patients with cancer probably didn't bother me anymore. I told them that the day that happened would be the day I would hang up my white coat. Now that I am retired I can tell you that it never stopped bothering me.

Communicating with Physicians

"Your ability to communicate is an important tool in your pursuit of your goal"
Les Brown

My father was a family doctor in Brooklyn and relayed an incident to me about a well-trained neurologist who opened a consulting practice in his hospital. In the beginning he walked around with his 'nose in the air', acting superior to the family physicians. After six months, when referrals were not coming as quickly as he hoped, he began to say "Good morning, Dr. Gilbert" when he passed him in the hall.

Communicating with other physicians is an important skill to master. Some primary care doctors are intimidated by cancer and hesitate to talk directly with the radiation oncologists. I always tried to be collegial and supportive in reaching out to my fellow physicians. I made a special effort to make myself available for phone calls from physicians who were asking for advice. I looked forward to these conversations and I never failed to thank them for calling. I considered it the ultimate compliment when a peer sought my counsel. I also built my schedule around physically attending the local tumor conferences. I made an effort to know the doctor's names and to chat with them during these visits. This relationship made it much easier for them to call me and I truly enjoyed the camaraderie. In fact, when the word was out that I was retiring, a couple of surgeons asked if they could still contact me occasionally to discuss cases.

Patients are often concerned about whether they should stay in their local hospital for cancer surgery or if they should go to the large referral center. When appropriate, I went out of my way to reassure them that they were receiving excellent care from their local doctors. An example of this is a patient who had a lumpectomy for breast cancer by her local surgeon, Dr.

67

Gordon Paine at Pen Bay Medical Center. She had a beautiful cosmetic result from the lumpectomy and I had to search for the scar. I told her that when she next saw Dr. Paine to tell him that Dr. Gilbert admired his work. A month later at the local tumor board, Gordon came over to me with a smile and said he got my message.

One experience showed me that good doctor to doctor communication is very similar to a good doctor to patient relationship. To appreciate the clinical situation one must realize that management of cancer is continuously evolving and some excellent cancer center's treatment protocols may differ from those of others. Bulky head and neck (H&N) cancer is an example. Radiotherapy alone was used at the Mass General by my mentor, CC Wang, who was regarded as a top H &N radiation oncologist. Across the city at the Dana Farber Cancer Center however, they did studies on combining chemo and RT and had improved tumor control but at a heavy cost in patient morbidity. The combination caused increased inflammation of the mucous lining of the mouth and throat and marked difficulty in swallowing. This was treated aggressively with pain medication and a feeding tube to maintain nutrition in more than half of the patients. At Maine Med we used combined chemo and RT for these patients, influenced by our medical oncologist, Tom Ervin who was trained at the Dana Farber and had a special interest in H & N tumors.

A young Ear, Nose and Throat (ENT) surgeon opened an office in Brunswick. He was very well trained, an excellent surgeon and a caring physician. I had a good relationship with him since I was then spending most of my clinical time in our Bath facility, but he was not known to my partners, who spent most of their time in the Portland area. He referred a patient with a large bulky head and neck tumor to our department for treatment and one of my partners saw him. My partner recommended combining radiotherapy with chemotherapy and referred the patient to a medical oncologist for evaluation and treatment. When the referring surgeon heard about using chemo he called my partner and told him that he was trained to treat this lesion with RT alone since the results of combined treatment did not justify the increased morbidity associated with the use of both modalities. My partner was in the middle of a busy clinic with three patients waiting for him and he told the surgeon that recent studies showed a significant benefit from combined treatment and our ENT Tumor team agreed to use it as our standard. When the referring doctor further challenged him, my partner told him that he was very busy in the clinic and could not discuss it any further at that time.

A few minutes later the surgeon called me. He was very upset and wanted me to get involved with the decision of which treatment to use. I told him that I would review the chart and discuss it with my partner. The patient did indeed have a large, locally advanced cancer and I felt that the combined treatment was justified. I called the surgeon and asked if he would be willing to meet with me to discuss the management of this patient and I suggested that we invite the other two ENT surgeons from the Brunswick area as well as the two local medical oncologists. He agreed and I contacted the four other doctors and arranged a meeting at Mid Coast Hospital for the following week. A few days before the meeting I sent each copies of six pertinent journal articles that described the results of combined therapy for this disease. Everyone read the articles and we had an excellent discussion. At the end of the meeting we all agreed that the positive results did justify the use of combined therapy and the added significant morbidity could be managed with aggressive supportive care in almost all patients.

While all physicians want to offer the very best care for their patients, sometimes management protocols do differ significantly from one center to another and occasionally from one physician to another. There is often not one best approach. The physician should treat his colleague as he would want to be treated, with respect and solid information and data to justify the recommendation.

The multiple Tumor Boards that our staff attended, both at Maine Med and at our referring hospitals, were in-house professional educational meetings centered around presenting and discussing interesting current cases. They were staffed by pathologists, diagnostic radiologists, all the involved clinical specialists and the general medical staff. These sessions provided us with an excellent opportunity to discuss with our fellow physicians the management of patients and how RT could enhance the results of surgery and chemotherapy. These meetings enhanced a good working relationship with our colleagues and allowed us to establish common guidelines and protocols that we all felt were warranted by the current literature.

NETWORKING WITH OTHER PHYSICIANS

When I was at the Mass General, the staff did not know the radiation oncologists in Maine which concerned them about the quality of care for their patients. If they saw a patient from Maine or another part of Northern New England that person was often encouraged to stay in Boston to receive sophisticated radiotherapy.

An important part of building a practice was networking to meet with other physicians in oncology and to earn their respect and friendship. I was very active in the New England Society for Radiation Oncology (NESRO) which consisted of radiation oncologists from all six New England states. I was Secretary of this organization for several years and then President. When it was thriving we had fifty to seventy-five radiation oncologists attending its four regional meetings each year. In 1975, while still at the Mass General, I and a carload of my colleagues attended a NESRO meeting held at Maine Medical's new radiotherapy department and I was very impressed with the facility. This organization provided us with an opportunity to get to know and socialize with our counterparts in other cities and that made it very easy to refer patients back and forth and to discuss common issues.

Another organization that I was active in was the New England Cancer Society. This group consisted of physicians who dealt with cancer including surgeons, medical, radiation, pediatric, and gynecological oncologists as well as pathologists, ENT and so on. I was Secretary-Treasurer of this organization for several years and enjoyed their camaraderie and discussing treatment options with other specialists. Every couple of years a trip to Europe was arranged to visit some major cancer centers and those of us who went enjoyed an interesting meeting and fascinating tours organized by our hosts.

I initiated a Maine Radiation Oncology group and invited the radiation oncologists from the other four centers to meet for dinner in Augusta to discuss challenging cases. It gave us a chance to get to know one another and was also an opportunity to inform our colleagues of our current protocols. As a result of presentations at these meetings, we had referrals to Chris Seitz for his radioactive implants and to Maine Med's Intra-Operative Radiotherapy program for pancreatic cancers. Unfortunately all three of these regional organizations eventually dried up due to lack of interest and competing educational meetings.

BREAST CANCER PATIENTS

> "IF YOU HAVE A FRIEND OR FAMILY MEMBER
> WITH BREAST CANCER, TRY NOT TO LOOK AT HER
> WITH 'SAD EYES'. TREAT HER LIKE YOU ALWAYS
> DID; JUST SHOW A LITTLE EXTRA LOVE."
> HODA KOTB

The following three patients with breast cancer had unusual courses which demonstrate the variation and unpredictability of this disease.

A sixty-three year old lady with an early left breast cancer was treated with a mastectomy. The margins were clear and the nodes were negative. After surgery she was seen in Boston and started on Tamoxifen, a drug that blocks the estrogen effect on the breast cancer. She returned to Maine and her family physician renewed her prescriptions every six months. After he retired the patient was seen by a new physician who while reviewing her meds noted that she had been on Tamoxifen for fifteen years. He told her that five years is the recommended length of time to be on the drug and he took her off of it. Three years later, eighteen years after her mastectomy, she developed an ulcerating lesion in the mid-portion of her mastectomy incision. The biopsy revealed recurrent breast cancer, the lesion was resected and the left chest wall was irradiated. At the end of her six weeks of radiotherapy, she was restarted on Tamoxifen. This eighty-one year old, four feet eleven inch lady looked me straight in the eye, shook her finger in my face and said "God help the next doctor who tries to take me off of Tamoxifen". She had no evidence of active disease for the three years I followed her. I have no doubt she continued on the drug for the remainder of her life.

Tamoxifen has been around for over twenty years and has been shown to reduce recurrences at five years in Estrogen Receptor positive breast cancer patients by 25%. The original studies tested two groups. Half took the drug for five years and others did a ten year course. There was no signifi-cant survival difference in the two groups so five years became the recom-mended regimen. Fifteen year follow-up studies do indicate however, that five years on Tamoxifen will have a 10% long term tumor control rate and an additional 15 % of the total will have a recurrence after Tamoxifen is stopped at five years. Continuing hormonal therapy past five years with Tamoxifen or the Aromatase Inhibitors (Arimidex or Femora) may provide a longer remission but its effect on cure rate is uncertain. There are always some unfortunate patients who are destined to recur when the hormonal resistant cells take over.

A post-menopausal woman with an early breast cancer was treated with a lumpectomy, chemotherapy, radiotherapy and a five year course of Tamoxi-fen. She did well and had no evidence of recurrence. Seventeen years after her tumor was first treated she was admitted to the hospital with a signif-icant septicemia. She had hypotension, renal failure, and GI bleeding. She was treated in the Intensive Care Unit for a four week period and finally stabilized and was discharged. A month after discharge she was seen for bone pain. A bone scan revealed wide spread bone metastases and biopsy revealed metastatic breast cancer. Studies have shown that breast cancer cells can be found in the peripheral blood and in bone marrow even in early cancer. It is believed that these cells can be dormant for years but can grow and metastasize if the patient's immune system falters, which is apparent-ly what happened as a result of her septicemia. Fortunately this is a rare occurrence.

About twenty years ago I was on call for a three day holiday weekend. On Friday afternoon I received a telephone call from a referring physician that a lady from the mid-coast area had a newly diagnosed left breast cancer that had metastasized to an upper thoracic vertebral body. She was having weakness in her legs and was unable to walk. This suggested that the tumor was pressing on the spinal cord making it a radiotherapeutic emergency requiring immediate treatment. She was given steroids to try to reduce the pressure on her spine and was transferred to our hospital. On examination she had a large, neglected breast cancer that practically replaced her left breast and it was ulcerated and infected. The CT scan revealed a mass in the upper thoracic spine that was pressing on the spinal cord. I brought her down to our department and gave her the first of ten radiation treatments starting with a larger than usual dose in order to reduce the size of the tumor as quickly as possible before permanent damage to the spinal cord occurred. We treated her Friday night, and daily throughout the three day weekend. She was also treated with antibiotics for her infected breast and was started on systemic hormonal therapy to treat the tumor. Workup revealed no other gross tumor involvement. On Tuesday the patient had full strength in her legs and was walking. She also responded to the hormonal therapy and the breast lesion responded well enough to permit a cleansing mastectomy about six weeks later. After she healed from her surgery I treated the left chest wall to prevent any local recurrence. She continued on hormonal therapy and was alive without any evidence of tumor activity eight years later when I discharged her from my follow-up care. Long term control of metastatic disease with hormones can last for twenty years or more.

ANN MURRAY PAIGE

> **"WE HAVE ABSOLUTELY NO CONTROL OVER WHAT HAPPENS TO US IN LIFE BUT WHAT WE HAVE PARAMOUNT CONTROL OVER IS HOW WE RESPOND TO THOSE EVENTS."**
>
> VIKTOR FRANKL

Ann Murray Paige was one of the most interesting and likable patients I have ever treated. I knew of her from her excellent work as a reporter and anchor on WCSH TV. She was referred to me in 2004 for irradiation to the chest wall to treat her breast cancer after she had her mastectomies. When she came to my office for the consultation, accompanied by her sister-in-law, Linda Pattillo, she asked if she could tape our discussion. I have had several patients pull out their tape recorder before, but I was a bit taken back when Linda pulled out a video camera and began to check the lighting in the room. When I was given the go ahead to start talking I was at first very conscious of the camera in my face; however after a few minutes the discussion flowed with ease. As an experienced reporter, Ann asked good questions, took notes and had a good understanding of what to expect from radiotherapy. She sailed through radiation and our staff and Ann had a good warm relationship. My wife and I were pleased to attend the showing of her documentary, *Breast Cancer Diaries* in Waterville several months after the completion of her treatments. Unfortunately some of my best scenes wound up on the editor's floor. She did well for the couple of years that I followed her and I was saddened to learn that the tumor had metastasized to her lung during her sixth year of follow-up in 2009, in California. Over the following five year period her liver and brain became involved. Throughout her ordeal she continued to remind us through her writing "that all is not lost when things aren't going right". She spoke at cancer events, and wrote several books, including one for children who are dealing with their mother's breast cancer, all while attending spinning and yoga classes and working out with a trainer to help improve her lung capacity. She wrote *In the Pink*, her one-woman show, letting high school kids know that "the world can be tough but they can be tougher, if we all stick together". She self-published *Pink Tips* and started a non-profit called Project Pink whose mission is to distribute a copy of *Pink Tips* to every newly diagnosed breast cancer patient across the country and one day, around the world.

At a medical conference at MIT, a physician asked how they could make their oncologic practice better. She answered, "I guess my advice to all medical people is this: to make your practice better, every time you open that patient door to see another frightened face on the other side, whisper to yourself 'there but for the Grace of God go I.' It's compassion that will make us all feel better as we fight for our lives and you try to smother this world cancer beast—once and for all". She valiantly fought her disease and continued to share her experiences with her friends on the web right up until her death in March of 2014. If you are ever in need of inspiration, google Ann Murray Paige and read her blogs. We can all learn from her as she knew how to keep that glass half full and how to die living. Ann is yet another reminder of how much more work we need to do to conquer this awful and unpredictable disease.

Hodgkin's Disease

> "You may not control all the events that happen to you, but you can decide not to be reduced by them." Maya Angelou

Hodgkin's disease is a malignant tumor of the lymph system that usually spreads from one nodal group to another in a predicable fashion. It occurs most often in young adults, between the ages of fifteen to forty, but is also seen in those over fifty-five with a less predictable mode of spread. It was a lethal disease in the early twentieth century but the work of Dr. Henry Kaplan at Stanford and others took advantage of the predicable spread of the disease and successfully controlled the majority of young patients with radiotherapy. During the second half of the twentieth century, the research concentrated on reducing the extent of treatment to avoid long term side effects without reducing the effectiveness of the treatment.

A forty year old woman presented in 1980 with a large mediastinal mass that was diagnosed as Hodgkin's disease, and was staged as IIA since it also involved the supraclavicular nodes. She was treated by the local medical oncologist with MOPP chemotherapy for six cycles. She had a complete response but recurred after the last chemo dose. She was referred to the Dana Farber Cancer Center and was started on the English MOPP regimen. Unfortunately the tumor started to grow aggressively during the second cycle. Dr. Canellis from DFCC referred the patient to us for radiotherapy. At referral she had a significantly enlarged mediastinal mass. The RT portal encompassed all of her known tumor and included major portions of her lungs and upper heart. She had already received significant doses of Adriamycin, which affects the heart, and Bleomycin, which affects the lung. I had a frank discussion with the patient telling her that the tumor was aggressive and may not respond well to radiotherapy and that I would have to include significant portions of her heart and lungs which may cause permanent harmful effects. She agreed that we did not have many options and she wanted to proceed with the treatment. She tolerated it well and all tumors cleared. I followed her for ten years and she did not recur or develop significant after effects. When I retired in 2008, she came to an open house that Pen Bay Medical Center held in my honor. At my final Tumor Board, the President of Pen Bay, Roy Hutchins, told the group that she said that I saved her life. My answer to that comment was that if I take credit for the ones that did well, I would have to take the blame for the ones that didn't. I thus chose not to accept credit for either. This case also demonstrates the importance of appreciating what other modalities can contribute to the patient. Dr. Canellis, a world renowned medical oncologist realized that chemo was not working and rather than try different drugs referred the patient for radiotherapy.

At a tumor conference a few years ago they presented a young patient with Hodgkin's. I commented that in my first decade of practice I loved to treat these patients because the cure rate was so high. As the years passed I saw that the treatment could lead to long term problems and my enthusiasm for treating these patients waned. The following are two examples of long term adverse effects associated with oncologic management.

The father of a young woman I had treated for Hodgkin's disease, earlier in my career, was referred to me with early stage prostate cancer. She did very well and was discharged after five years of follow-up. Her father told me that she was diagnosed with breast cancer at the age of forty and eventually died from that tumor. Young women who receive radiotherapy for Hodgkin's are at higher risk to develop breast cancer. He assured me that she continued with close medical surveillance as advised but she still failed.

I came across a woman at a social event about twenty years after I treated her for Hodgkin's disease and complimented her on how great she looked. She informed me that she was doing well but did need surgery for thyroid cancer which was successful.

One of the great challenges of oncology is 'not knowing what we don't know'. Many of the significant after effects of cancer treatment are not appreciated until fifteen to twenty years later. The above two patients are examples from our treatment of Hodgkin's. Other examples include the radiotherapy of breast cancer with tangential, opposed fields. At the Mass General I was taught to include the whole bed of the breast. With the machines used at that time, that necessitated treating a portion of the heart when irradiating the left side. Twenty years later we found that women who had significant heart irradiation developed a higher rate of cardiac difficulties. Today, with modern radiotherapy machines, we are able to avoid as much cardiac exposure as possible.

Another example involves the chemo drug Adriamycin. This was the primary drug used for most chemo regimens for breast cancer. It was known that this drug could injure the heart but it was generally accepted that if the total dose of the drug was limited, then cardiac damage was not a problem. Fifteen years later women who received the lower dose of Adria still developed a higher incidence of cardiac problems.

One of the advantages of a long career is what we learn from experience. What you thought you knew for sure sometimes does not always stand up to the test of time. In our rush to market new drugs, we forget that what we don't know can hurt us.

PROSTATE CANCER

"WE CURE A LOT OF PATIENTS WHO DO NOT
NEED TO BE CURED, AND WE TREAT A LOT OF
MEN WHO WE CANNOT CURE."
DR. WILLET WHITMORE, M.D.

Today, prostate cancer is by far the most commonly diagnosed cancer in American males. It more than doubles the second most commonly diagnosed cancer, which is lung. Before the Prostate Specific Antigen (PSA) blood marker was introduced in the early 1980's, only seventy thousand U.S. men were diagnosed each year and about 50%, or thirty-five thousand died annually. After PSA screening, up to three hundred thousand were identified on a yearly basis but the absolute death rate changed very little. The 'cure rate' skyrocketed since so many asymptomatic men, with tumors that were not life threatening were now being diagnosed and treated. Autopsy studies have taught us that 15% of men over the age of sixty who died of other causes will be found to have incidental prostate cancer, 33% will be found in those over seventy, and 50% will be found in those over eighty. Thus prostate cancer is a 'disease' of aging and the great majority of men who are diagnosed with it would be better off NOT knowing since treatment would not buy them improvement in their health or longevity. Even though over 75% of those diagnosed have incidental prostate cancer it cannot be ignored entirely, since it is the second leading cause of cancer death in U.S. males. The latest American Cancer Society numbers tell us that in 2014, 84,930 men died of lung cancer, 29,480 died of prostate cancer and 26,270 from colo-rectal cancer.

Today there is controversy concerning whether PSA screening is beneficial. If we gave definitive surgery or radiotherapy every time we diagnosed an early, low grade prostate cancer, then more patients would suffer from treatment, including early death then would benefit from it. I have had patients who died from a heart attack the night of prostatectomy and others who had strokes, MI's, and fistulas from the bladder to the colon in the post-op period. Both surgery and radiotherapy can cause morbidity with the rectum and bladder, as well as decreased potency. I strongly believe in the benefits of PSA screening and will continue to have my own drawn each year. Since I have never smoked, prostate cancer would be the number one cancer threat for me. If only those patients with intermediate or high risk disease were treated and the majority with low risk cancer was followed closely, then PSA screening would lead to curing some with early stage life threatening disease but minimize the unnecessary morbidity associated with treatment of incidental tumors.

Two patients illustrate issues associated with prostate screening. Both men were sixty-eight years old. One was in excellent general health and had a PSA of 3.8 four years before. Less than 4 is normal for his age. His doctor told him that the PSA was borderline high and that he should return in a year to have it repeated. He returned after a four year hiatus and his PSA was 15 and his biopsy showed a Gleason score of 9 out of 10, which is a high risk. After tests showed there was no evidence that the tumor had spread, he was treated with anti-androgen hormonal therapy and local radiotherapy. This man would have benefited from close follow-up of his PSA since treatment for his life threatening tumor could have started two or three years sooner.

The other sixty-eight year old patient, who I evaluated on the same day, had been followed with annual PSA's and when his PSA changed from 1.5 to 2.0 he was advised to have a needle biopsy. The biopsy showed two of twelve cores to be positive for low grade cancer. The urologist recommended surgery but changed his mind when he found out that he had previous surgical correction of an abdominal aortic aneurysm, which made the prostate surgery more difficult. He then referred the patient for radiotherapy. I found that the patient continued to smoke and had related vascular changes, not only in the aorta but in his legs and in addition had a diagnosis of coronary artery disease. I reassured him that his prostate cancer was low risk and that he did not need to have treatment at this time but would be followed closely with PSA's. If there was a progression of the prostate cancer we could always give treatment but we can't take it back. I also told him that stopping smoking would do a lot more to prolong his life than treating his prostate.

HORMONAL THERAPY

Prostate cancer is very sensitive to hormonal therapy. The only other tumor that is as sensitive to hormones is breast cancers that are positive for Estrogen receptors. About 95 to 98% of prostate cancer cells need Androgen stimulation to live. It is dramatic when a patient presents with widespread, advanced prostate cancer with painful metastases and a PSA in the hundreds. When this occurs they can be given anti-androgen therapy and the PSA will often come down to negligible levels, the pain clears and the patient goes into remission from months to a couple of years. The reason why it is not a cure is that the 2 to 5% of the cell population that is not dependent on Androgen stimulation takes over and patients eventually succumb from the hormone resistant cells. The remission from hormone therapy usually lasts about two to three years. The current treatment for resistant cells is chemotherapy and/or local palliative radiotherapy but new drugs are being introduced which will hopefully be more effective.

The following are two patients who demonstrated the unpredictability of this disease. I treated a seventy-two year old man in the late 1970's with a nodule on his prostate that proved to be cancerous. This was before the introduction of the PSA test so that patients were diagnosed either clinically, with symptoms of bone metastasis, urinary obstruction due to a large tumor mass in the prostate or a palpable nodule on rectal exam. A few lucky patients were diagnosed early when they had a Trans Urethral Resection (TUR) for urinary obstruction and the pathological evaluation of the removed chips showed prostate cancer. Most patients were diagnosed at a later stage and 50% died from their tumor. My patient was treated with external beam radiotherapy. He tolerated his initial four weeks of treatment well and then I noticed a palpable left supraclavicular node. I had that biopsied and it proved to be metastatic prostate cancer. His radiotherapy was discontinued after five of seven planned weeks and the urologist did a bilateral orchiectomy (removing the testicles), which was the hormone treatment of the day. This was before anti-androgen drugs were available. Over the next few weeks the palpable supraclavicular node and the nodule on the prostate both regressed. I followed him for the next twenty years and the tumor never returned. I discharged him from follow-up when he was ninety-two years old with no evidence of tumor. As I stated above, the average duration of hormonal remission is two to three years but there are occasional patients on both ends of the bell curve. This patient apparently had all of his cancer cells dependent on Androgen stimulation and when we removed the hormone, all the cells died.

The other patient was one of the strangest cases of prostate cancer I ever treated. This man was in his late sixties when he presented with an advanced local prostate malignancy. He had a hard lumpy prostate that appeared to be attached to the pelvic sidewalls by palpation. His PSA was elevated at 35 and his biopsy revealed a Gleason score of 10 out of 10. His risk for having extensive disease was very high but the CT scan of the abdomen and pelvis and the bone scan were all negative for tumor. I met with him and told him that he had advanced local disease that was not operable but we could treat him first with androgen hormone suppression therapy and then evaluate him for possible radiotherapy a few months later if no distant disease was evident. He told me that his son lived in North Carolina and that he was able to get an appointment with the Chief of Urology at one of the Universities in that area. I told him that the urologist he was scheduled to see was very famous but would not touch him with a ten foot pole. A week later he called to tell me that he had his consultation and was scheduled for a prostatectomy. I told him that that professor was a smart man and may know something I don't but if it was anybody else I would tell him to run and get a third opinion. The patient had his prostatectomy and indeed the Gleason score was 10 and the tumor extended outside the capsule and the surgical margins were positive. A couple of months after surgery his PSA came down to 1.5 but then started climbing, reaching 3.5 about six month's post-op.

I started him on my original plan of hormone suppression therapy and two months later I gave him radiation therapy to the prostatic bed and surrounding areas. The patient tolerated his treatments well and continued on hormone suppression for three years with a PSA of 0. I then stopped his hormone suppression and nervously followed his PSA. It remained at 0 for the next two years and then, six years after irradiation, the PSA climbed unexpectedly to 6. He was restarted on hormone suppression and followed by medical oncology. I know he did well for two years but was then lost to my follow-up when he moved away from Maine.

POST PROSTATECTOMY RECURRENCE

After the introduction of PSA screening, the incidence of prostatectomy increased significantly since the great majority of tumors were limited to the prostate itself. We then started to see a significant number of patients who were found to have tumor at the margins of resection. Only 50% of those with positive margins developed a local recurrence, manifested by a slow rise of the PSA from negligible to measureable. Several studies showed that radiotherapy to the surgical area of these patients could destroy the remaining tumor cells. The key was to initiate RT early enough before the tumor had a chance to spread beyond the tumor bed. Three international randomized studies showed that any patients with positive margins following prostatectomy had a significant cure rate with RT when compared to the control group that was not irradiated. These studies did not wait for measureable PSA recurrence.

In my practice, those patients who had significant, high risk local disease left behind after surgery were treated as soon as they recuperated and I did not wait for measureable PSA. I was concerned, however that treating all the patients with positive surgical margins would lead to giving RT to the 50% of patients who were not destined to fail. In those patients with minimal microscopic positive margins, I waited until I could document PSA recurrence before starting treatment. This provided an important benefit in that I hoped to avoid treating patients who were not destined to recur. By waiting at least a couple of months after surgery, I also allowed the patient to fully recover and regain full control of his bladder function.

My concern was that I did not want to wait too long and lose a chance of salvaging a cure. Consequently I studied all the patients I treated after prostatectomy and gathered information on sixty of them over a couple of years. My criteria were three fold. Their PSA prior to treatment had to be less than 20, there needed to be minimal residual disease after surgery and the PSA prior to RT had to be less than 1. Twenty of them fit these criteria. Of the twenty, eighteen were cured with a non-measurable PSA that persisted. One patient was referred six months after surgery with a PSA of 0.6. His tumor was irradiated and had no measureable PSA for four years. Measured again at four and a half years it stood at 0.4. Despite prolonging his remission by almost five years, the patient outcome was counted as a failure of treatment. The remaining patient in my series had a continued increase in his PSA despite his course of radiotherapy to the surgical site and presented with distant metastasis several months later.

My study convinced me that salvage post-prostatectomy could be safely delayed in patients with minimal residual disease until measurable PSA is detected. I personally started using a level of 0.3 as my trigger to avoid losing any patients to disseminated disease. A couple of years after my unpublished study there was a national discussion about whether it was prudent to delay salvage prostate radiotherapy. The following letter, outlines a protocol I had been using with my own patients, and before submitting it to the International Journal of Radiation Oncology, I shared it with my friend and colleague, Anthony Zeitman at Mass General. He is one of the leading experts on prostate radiation oncology and also happens to be Editor-in-Chief of the Journal. He wrote back that he agreed with my letter but the decision on whether it would be published would be left to the Opinion Page Editor.

Letter to the Editor

International Journal of Radiation Oncology, Biology, Physics

Dr. King's editorial on "Adjuvant radiotherapy after prostatectomy: Does waiting for a detectable prostate-specific antigen level make sense?" was well done and thought provoking.

In review of the non-irradiated control arms of the three quoted studies, EORTC 22911, SWOG 8794, and ARO 96-02, approximately 50% of truly adjuvant patients who do not receive RT are not destined to fail. In the arms receiving adjuvant RT the 5-year biochemical PSA relapse-free was 72 to 77% and thus a tumor control rate of approximately 25% better than those who did not receive RT.

My interpretation of the data is that the major cause of the increasing recurrence rate seen when the PSA increases from non-detectable to 0.5 is the elimination of patients who are not destined to fail. I do not believe it is due to progression of tumor to a non-curable stage.

The PSA level that would eliminate most of those who are destined not to fail can be easily determined by reviewing the PSA data on the control arms of the three studies. I would predict that a PSA value in the range from 0.3 to 0.5 would eliminate most of those patients who will not benefit from RT.

As we await the results of a possible prospective, randomized study, I would feel comfortable offering active surveillance to all post-prostatectomy cancer patients who have minimal residual tumor, obtaining a PSA every two to three months and then recommending salvage RT when the PSA reaches 0.3. This protocol would offer the following benefits:

1. *Eliminate approximately 50% of the patients who will not benefit from RT.*

2. *Provide additional time before commencement of RT so that the urinary sphincter can fully recover from surgery. This should reduce the incidence of incontinence.*

3. *Allow the urethral anastomosis more time to mature and thus reduce the risk of post-RT stricture.*

This protocol will provide the benefits to those patients who need post-prostatectomy RT and would minimize the harm to those who do not.

Stuart Gilbert, M.D.

(The letter was not published but I used this protocol for the patients that I treated and had good results.)

CLINICAL PROJECTS IN MAINE

"RESEARCH IS FORMALIZED CUROSITY. IT IS
POKING AND PRYING WITH A PURPOSE."
ZORA NEALE HURSTON

During my time at the Mass General and at Maine Med, I was involved with several clinical research projects that I considered a significant part of my clinical responsibilities. It is important to evaluate our results for clinical quality control and to question whether current protocols were accomplishing our goals. In the previous chapter I described my review of our results with post-operative PSA recurrence of prostate cancer. The following are other examples of these projects.

Shortly after I arrived in Maine I had lunch with a pathologist, Joe Fanning, in the doctor's cafeteria. He had just finished a long ENT operation where the surgeon was trying to get clear surgical margins. He did six frozen sections, each taking twenty to thirty minutes, until the surgeon was satisfied that there was no cancer in the surrounding tissue. Joe asked me if all these frozen sections really made a difference. I told him I didn't know but if he could pull all the head and neck cases from the previous year that had initial positive margins but were cleared eventually, I would try to see if we could come up with an answer. He gave me the pathology reports on five patients who were operated on in 1975 who fit our criteria. Four of the five had eventual clear surgical margins and no post-operative radiotherapy. They all failed locally despite the additional surgery. The fifth patient had pre-operative radiotherapy and had no recurrence. The rational for pre-op RT is to reduce the size of the tumor and injure it to the point that the residual tumor is less able to form new colonies. My conclusion from our small sample was that once the tumor is cut through, it could still seed into the wound and pre- or post-operative RT could be helpful in preventing recurrence. I also told Dr. Fanning that if we had residents and clerical support we could pull cases from the last ten years and may have a paper to publish. That never happened. I did present the results from this small sample to the ENT Tumor Conference.

My next project was my only major, published paper which involved a retrospective analysis of rectal cancer. See pages 27 and 28 for further details on this study. From this project I developed an excellent respect for and relationship with the Tumor Registry professionals at Maine Med. Their job is to gather data on the cancer patients and they are pleased when that information is used in a clinically useful manner. I also made myself available to them when they needed a doctor's assistance in assigning the proper stage for a tumor or when they had difficulty extracting data from a chart.

One of the projects I did with the Tumor Registrars concerned early stage lung cancers that were not resected. These tumors were slow growing nodules found on a chest CT scan. They were not operated on because either the patient's general health and lung reserve was so compromised that the surgeon felt the risk of surgery was too great or because a few patients refused to have surgery. It is tempting to treat these lesions with radiotherapy alone but I was not convinced that these sick patients could tolerate the treatment or that there would be meaningful prolongation of life. With the help of tumor registry we gathered information on sixty patients with non-small cell lung cancers that measured less than 3 cm. in diameter and who were treated with radiotherapy alone from 1996 to 2003. Pathology confirmation was obtained in two thirds of the patients and the remainder showed growth on subsequent scans. Seventeen percent were over the age of eighty-five years and 31% were older than eighty. Only 13% were younger than sixty-five years. The two year survival was 67%. At three years it was 46% and at four and one half years it was 32%. Since many of these patients were on nasal oxygen and had advanced co-morbidities, I was impressed with these results. The other important question was whether these patients could tolerate the treatment. I was delighted to find out that only one died within nine months of treatment and that was at three months. These results were published in Maine Med's Annual Cancer report and were presented at the hospital's Lung Tumor Conference.

Early in my career at Mass General, we treated unresectable pancreatic cancers with Intraoperative Radiotherapy (IORT). In order to control these tumors high doses of irradiation were required but the surrounding area contained vital structures, such as the liver, kidneys, spinal cord, bowel and stomach that could be damaged by such doses. IORT involves taking the patient to the operating room and exposing the pancreatic tumor. If the tumor is indeed localized then the wound is covered with sterile drapes and then the patient is taken from the OR, under anesthesia, to the radiotherapy suite. There the tumor is exposed and a sterile tube that is attached to the radiotherapy head is aimed at the tumor. High dose localized irradiation could then be delivered with other vital structures protected. Between 1984 and 1986 we successfully did eighteen cases without any problems. Sixteen other patients were scheduled for IORT but were aborted when the tumor was found to have spread. No patient encountered any infection or other complication of the procedure and all left the hospital as would be expected after surgery alone. None of these patients were cured but they had significant pain control. Several major cancer centers reported similar results. Since it did not lead to cure and there were other available methods to control pain, it was felt that the procedure was not warranted and we stopped using it. This technique was a huge multi-departmental project. The OR had to supply needed equipment to the RT facility, security had to secure the halls and elevator needed for transportation and housekeeping scrubbed down the radiotherapy room to make it as sterile as possible. In addition, our daily schedule on that machine had to be cleared for a two hour period. I was very impressed how all the different departments rallied to make this complicated procedure run as smoothly as it did.

I believe a major function of an excellent department is to review their results and make sure they are achieving the best outcomes possible. Tumor Registries and good computerized records will facilitate success. In an era of compensation based on quality of patient care, all these 'tools' will be vital to physicians, hospitals and patients alike.

JACK GIBSON'S PHILANTHROPY

In 1988 and 1989 I took care of Susan Gibson who was always accompanied by her devoted husband. She had a cancer that had spread to her bones causing multiple episodes of painful metastases that required several courses of palliative radiotherapy. We spent much time discussing her disease and what we were going to do to try to alleviate her symptoms. The patient and her husband were always kind and considerate of the staff and very appreciative of the efforts our Department made to help her. Shortly after she passed away I received the following letter from her husband.

May 1, 1989

Dear Dr. Gilbert,

I wish to thank you, your nursing staff and therapists for the kind care and attention given to Susan during her ordeal. The professionalism, love and support that is in abundance in the Radiology Department did not go unnoticed. Susan was so fortunate to have had such good people in attendance during her illness. I wish the very best to those whom assisted her.

Sincerely,

Marshall (Jack) Gibson

I responded with the following letter:

May 5, 1989

Dear Jack,

Thank you for your very thoughtful letter.

It is said, that you can tell the true mettle of an individual only under the most adverse circumstances. Throughout her illness, both you and Susan always conducted yourselves in a very dignified manner. No matter how intense Susan's pain was, she always showed her appreciation and understanding to those who were caring for her. Many times I felt that Susan was trying to console me from my disappointment, in not being able to alleviate her pain. Susan and you earned my respect and the respect and admiration of all in our department.

Please accept my heartfelt sympathy in your loss. Having known Susan, I know how enormous that loss was.

If I can be of any further assistance in the future, please do not hesitate to contact me.

Sincerely,

Stuart Gilbert, M.D.

A month later I received a copy of a letter that Jack Gibson sent to the MMC's Development office. It was his first substantial annual gift to our Department.

Over the subsequent years Jack and I have enjoyed an occasional lunch together. In the late 1990's, he invited Carol and me to the 50th anniversary celebration of his road construction business. He started the business shortly after he returned from the war and it grew into a large company employing hundreds of workers. His party was at his company's facility and was attended by well over a thousand people. It was held on a beautiful summer day with lots of food, entertainment for adults and children and music. Jack proudly showed me the giant machinery that recycles old asphalt and the state of the art equipment that they use to build roads. I spent a lot of time speaking to his employees and others who knew him and I was repeatedly told how well Jack treated his employees. One attendee told me that he was hurt on the job and Jack looked in on him and gave him a light duty job until he was able to return to his regular work. He did not miss a single pay check. He also told me of another worker who became disabled and Jack found a job for his wife so that the household would still have a pay check coming in, along with the disability insurance. That afternoon convinced me that a major reason for the success of his company was the loyalty and affection that his employees had for him.

A few years later I was attending an Oncology Steering Committee meeting when Dr. Bob Hillman, the head of the cancer program, announced to the group that the husband of one of my patients donated $2 million to name the new inpatient oncology facility. That was the second largest gift that MMC ever received up to that time. I sent the following letter to Jack to thank him for his annual gift to our department.

February 7, 2003

Dear Jack,

Thank you for your continued support of the radiation therapy department. Your generous contribution will again be used to pro-vide our patients with extra comfort and services that the hospital usually does not provide such as educational books, tapes, candy in the jar, small gifts for our pediatric patients and so on. Those "little" touches send a huge signal of caring and compassion to our patients and their families.

Your philanthropy is particularly meaningful to me. In other cas-es, wealthy people can write a check and expect their generosity to buy them respect and admiration. On the other hand, if you never gave a penny, you would still be considered a generous compas-sionate and caring man who has beneficially touched the lives of many Mainers over your successful career. You have earned the respect and admiration of the community the hard way, not just by giving a check.

Maine Medical Center is very fortunate and honored to have its Oncology facility named after Susan and you.

With respect and admiration, I am

Yours very truly,

Stu

True to form, Jack Gibson has not only given the money to build the Oncology Floor, he has become involved in supporting the facility and its staff. He brought coffee and goodies on Sunday mornings for the staff and hosted a barbeque at his home in the summer for the staff and their families.

I was disappointed that MMC did not thank the staff of our department and tell them how much they appreciated the hospital benefitting from their good work. They should show the same appreciation to the staff as they do to donors from the community. An acknowledgment would have gone a long way to make the staff feel like a team player and give them ownership and responsibility for the hospital. When they had the ground breaking event that commenced construction I was not informed and wasn't in attendance. Jack called me afterwards to say that he was surprised that I was not there. When I explained why, he told me that he would make sure that I was involved with the opening ceremony. A couple of years later, the head of the MMC Development office ran into me at the Woodlands Club and said that Jack Gibson wants me to accompany him, Barbara and George Bush on the private tour of the Gibson Oncology Pavilion and the Barbara Bush Children's Hospital at the time of the dedication. I was honored.

CHRIS SEITZ

C hris Seitz was a fellow radiation oncologist who joined our group a couple of years after me. We practiced together for twenty-five years and shared many good times both in and outside of the hospital. He was a very adventurous individual who loved the outdoors. He entered endurance challenges such as runs up Pike's Peak and bike races up Mount Washington and loved to ski and ride his motorcycle. Tragically, in March of 2002, Chris was helicopter skiing with his two sons in British Columbia when he died in an avalanche. Fortunately no one else was injured. His wife Ann asked his partners to speak at his funeral. I gave the following eulogy at the filled to capacity Woodfords Congregational Church on March 24, 2002.

For the past twenty-five years I have had the privilege and pleasure to share my professional life with Chris Seitz. During that time, he was my consultant, confident, and great friend. He was also my partner for various business ventures. Fortunately, Chris and I kept our day jobs.

Today, I want to say a few words about Chris Seitz, the physician. Chris was the complete package. He was a superb and resourceful radiation oncologist who was able to introduce new techniques and perfect old ones. His expertise in radioactive implants was universally recognized throughout the region. In fact, any difficult implants from Lewiston to Presque Isle were referred to Chris.

He was an excellent physician with an extraordinary fund of knowledge. If any of our department's staff had a medical problem, almost always they would seek out Chris for advice and treatment. If that staff member needed to see a specialist, then Chris would be on the phone and arrange an expeditious appointment, just as if his own family member needed to be seen. Chris also took his responsibility to the community very seriously. He spoke at many cancer support groups, community meetings and was President of the local chapter of the American Cancer Society.

However the truest test or challenge to the physician caring for cancer patients is not only how they take care of the cancer, but more importantly, how they care for the family and the human being who is attached to that cancer. Chris combined his great knowledge and technical ability with a compassionate and caring heart of gold. Several of his patients refused to be discharged after being followed for four or five years after treatment, and insisted on seeing 'their' doctor once a year to make sure all was well. Chris was admired, loved and now mourned by hundreds of patients and their families whose lives he has touched over the past years.

Chris would want me to say at this time that the physician is only one member of a team that provides quality care in a compassionate manner. He would want me to thank the dedicated staffs at Maine Med and Presque Isle, most of whom are present today. Their outstanding efforts and loving care allowed him and all of us to provide the care and caring that we all are proud of.

Finally, I would like to share with you my favorite Chris Seitz story. He, especially in his youth, was a very competitive individual who loved to challenge himself to the limit. He ran marathons, ran a road race up Pike's Peak in Colorado, and entered the annual bike race up Mt. Washington. When he was a resident in radiology at Maine Med in 1975, he entered the Portland Boys Club five mile road race that is held every Patriot's Day. While at the starting line, a friend pointed out this petite, thin young girl and said it was John Gibbons' niece. John Gibbons was the Chief of Radiology and our boss. The race started and this girl matched Chris step for step. In the middle of the race she started pulling away from him and this macho guy was not going to let that happen so he stepped up his pace. In the final stretch, although complete-

ly exhausted, he put on a final sprint and beat her to the finish line. Later, he found out that this young high school senior was Joan Benoit who, nine years later, went on to win an Olympic gold medal in the marathon.

Ann, speaking for Chris' professional family, I want to tell you and your wonderful family, that we fully appreciate the enormity of your loss, and our thoughts, prayers and love are with you.

INTERESTING PATIENT SITUATIONS

STUDENT WITH LEUKEMIA

The treatment of childhood leukemia is one of the great advances of the last fifty years. When I was in medical school it was fatal in practically all cases and today it has a 90% cure rate.

The following vignette involved an eighth grader in the Cape Elizabeth Middle School who was a family friend. She was diagnosed with Acute Lymphoblastic Leukemia and was treated with multi-drug chemotherapy followed by consolidation low dose radiotherapy to the brain. As mentioned elsewhere in this book, the chemotherapy used at that time did not cross the blood-brain barrier so the concentration of chemo drugs that entered the brain was not high enough to eradicate every last leukemic cell. After the cancerous cells were cleared from the peripheral blood and bone marrow, the chemo would be stopped and almost all of the patients would then fail with recurrence in the brain that would in turn spread to the remainder of the body. Eventually, treatment included a low dose RT to eliminate persistent cells in the brain and with that change the cure rate rose to over 50%.

What made this young girl's treatment so memorable is that the Maine Children's Cancer Program at Maine Med made a special effort to keep these children in school and to involve the teachers and fellow students in their care. The nurses from the Program went to the school and gave an in-service to the teachers and discussed the plan of treatment and the expected side effects and how to handle them. They stressed how effective the current management was and that she had an excellent long-term prognosis. These nurses then stepped into the classroom to 'teach' her classmates about leukemia. They created a very real picture for those children, including her treatment and the real hope that she would be cured as a result of her chemo and radiation therapy. Students came to understand that their classmate would feel nauseous, tired, have a decreased appetite and lose her hair. Lots of questions were asked and answered in that classroom with the hope that their support would make her treatment and recovery just a bit easier.

Our patient went through her treatments with tremendous support from her school and friends. She did very well and returned to a full active life very quickly after completion of the therapy. I attended her graduation ceremony from Cape Elizabeth High School four years later and was moved when her classmates gave her a special award for her courage and spirit that helped to defeat her leukemia. There was then a prolonged standing ovation as she came forward to accept her award. I don't think there was a dry eye in the building.

The great lesson of this story is that a terrible tragedy can become an important teaching moment not only for the school but also for the whole community. Her classmates, who think they are invincible and will live forever learned that good health is precious and should not be taken for granted and a genuine word of encouragement and support can make a huge difference for those who are suffering.

DOCTOR AS JUDGE AND JURY

I treated a man in his late sixties who was estranged from his family and had a long history of alcohol and tobacco abuse. He was accompanied by a male friend who brought him in on a daily basis for the six weeks of radiotherapy to treat his lung cancer which had spread to the mediastinal nodes. He tolerated the course of treatment well and when he returned six weeks later for a follow-up the CT scan showed dramatic diminution of the tumor. I shared the results with my patient and his friend and told them I was very pleased with how he tolerated the treatments and how the tumor had responded. I gave him an appointment to come back in three months.

About one month later I received a call from a lawyer who informed me that the patient died suddenly a couple of weeks after I saw him and he and the opposing lawyer would like to meet with me. We met in my office and they explained that two days before his follow-up appointment my patient rewrote his will, leaving all his assets to his friend and nothing to his family. Two days after his appointment with me, he signed the Will in his lawyer's office. The family challenged the new Will stating that he was not competent at the time. The Judge ruled that since an unbiased physician examined him between the time he first saw the lawyer and the time that he signed it, then I should be the one to determine if he was or was not competent. I read my note of that day to the lawyers and told them that I discussed the findings on the CT scan with him and he fully understood them and showed no evidence of incompetence. The two lawyers thanked me and left. End of story and most likely the law suit.

TREATING A PRISONER

> **"STATE PRISONS ARE LARGE WAREHOUSES THAT SEPARATE THE PRISONER FROM SOCIETY WHICH LEAVES THEM FEELING DEHUMANIZED. ADD A DIAGNOSIS OF CANCER AND YOU FIND LITTLE HOPE LEFT IN A PRISONER'S LIFE."**
> MOIRA LACHANCE

A prisoner serving a life sentence for murder at the maximum security prison in Warren came to be my patient. At sixty-three years of age, he had been institutionalized since 1976. I recently learned from a Google search that he was convicted for killing a man in the 1970's. He was paroled briefly in the 1990's at which time he visited his mother in Florida. She reported to the police that he stole her car and a couple of days later her body was found. Her son was arrested in her car a couple of states away and had some blood stains on his clothes that matched the mother's blood type. Rather than try him for his mother's murder he was returned to the Maine prison for the remainder of his life term but this time without the chance of parole.

He had lung cancer with brain metastases and came in for daily treatments in shackles, accompanied by two guards. The staff and I treated him like any other patient. At the end of treatments he tearfully thanked me and the staff for giving him the dignity of treating him like a human being. He wrote the following note shortly before he passed away.

Ladies and Gentlemen,

I cannot find the correct words to thank you for treating me. You are all professional, courteous but most of all you cared. You looked beyond the prison guards and treated the man lying on the table. No matter how this goes for me, I will always remember you for your kindness and your gentleness.

Wishing you long and beautiful lives and may the winds always be at your back.

With all my heart, thank you!!

PERSONAL REVELATIONS

When the physician establishes a relationship with the patient as one who listens and cares, then the patient will be more open to share thoughts or concerns that they may never have mentioned to another individual.

I treated a fifty-five year old lady who had uterine cancer. Her hysterectomy specimen revealed that the tumor involved the lower uterine segment, near the surgical margin giving her a 10% risk of vaginal apex recurrence. To reduce this risk we inserted a plastic tube containing radioactive material into the lumen of her vagina and left it in place as an inpatient for approximately forty hours. This irradiated the vaginal apex to a depth of about one cm. sparing the rectum and bladder from significant irritation.

Today we can deliver the treatment as an outpatient using high dose rate sources.

At her follow up appointment four weeks later I told the patient that she healed well and could resume sexual intercourse or use a plastic dilator to prevent adhesions from forming in the vagina. She started to cry and when I asked her what was wrong, she told me that she and her husband were products of Catholic schools and after their fourth child was born fifteen years before, her husband said that they didn't need any more children and that was the last time they were intimate.

The Catholic Church taught that sexual relations between a husband and wife is for reproduction and the use of birth control, such as the pill, condoms and so on is a sin. With all due respect, I wonder if the rules would be different if they weren't made by elderly, white celibate men.

A Controlling Patient with Lung Cancer

A man in his early sixties presented with lung cancer that involved his mediastinal nodes. He had a personality that made him feel the need to be in control at all times. This played out throughout his entire treatment. He never appeared in clinic with any family member or friend. If someone drove him, they waited in the car, thus any reports about his condition or care were relayed by him to his family. His strong sense of self led him to suggest on a regular basis how we could improve our practice, his treatment and whatever else came to mind.

In time, he developed local and regional failure as well as distant metastases. For the last month of his life, his family set up a hospital bed in the living room and a different family member stayed with him during the night. On our last visit, three weeks before his death, he told me that during the previous Wednesday he could not catch his breath. He felt as if he was drowning in his own secretions. He said that his seventeen year old grandson stayed up with him all night and hovered over him, anxious to do whatever he could to give his grandfather some relief. The patient looked up at me and said "Doc that was the first time in my life that I ever felt loved." On his death bed, this frail, frightened man finally realized the value of loving and caring for another human being. It is sad to spend ones whole life with the strong feeling that to accept any kindness or help from others is a sign of weakness.

THE PERIOD OF SLEEPLESS NIGHTS

Several years ago, the topic for the guest speaker's lecture at our Spectrum Medical Group's Annual Meeting was "The Period of Sleepless Nights" which refers to the time between when a patient is told they have a problem to the time that it is addressed.

I had three experiences early in my career that made me very cognizant of this problem. The first was a man I had treated for an early stage lung cancer two years before and was doing well. He came in for a routine six month follow-up with a very sad and frightened look on his face. I asked him what was wrong and he pointed to his forearm and said "the cancer is back". I looked at it and told him that it was a benign cyst and nothing to worry about it. I then asked him when he first noticed it and thought it was a recurrence and he said that it was two months ago. Tragically he lived with the thought that the tumor had recurred for two full months. This was a 'teachable moment' for both my patient and me. I learned that patients should be encouraged to call with any concerns about symptoms. When dealing with cancer, there are no minor concerns. If there is a problem, then the sooner it is detected the more effective the treatment. On the other hand, if it is a false alarm, then the patient can be reassured and relieved of their anxiety.

Another patient completed her treatments for breast cancer. A couple of months later she called me from a pay phone outside of Disney World in Orlando. She was with her family and felt a supraclavicular node and was concerned that the tumor had recurred. I took the number of the pay phone (before cell phones there were pay phones) and told her I would call her right back. I then called the cancer center in Orlando and asked them to evaluate her. They agreed and I called her back with the information. Forty-five minutes later she called from the cancer center that all was clear.

Her vacation resumed without any more interruptions or anxiety.

My third experience occurred after the patient had passed away. I had treated Bill Hopkins, a middle aged man for a lung cancer. He was a fisherman and an English teacher and wrote a book about his illness called *Better than Dying.* Since he lived on North Haven Island off the mid coast of Maine, he stayed at his sister's house during the week. In his book, which was a journal about his battle with cancer, he wrote the following about taking a bone scan while he was undergoing radiotherapy to his chest.

"When the bone scan was over, I asked the girl if I might see, before I left, the pictures she had taken, and when she showed me the celluloid film, outlining me in black and white dots, I noticed a curious concentration of the dots in the area of my chest cancer, which is alarmingly huge, but I also noticed a similar concentration of the dots in my lower back, with which I have perpetually had problems for years. From this, I concluded that I had, as well, a big cancer in my lower back. And when I quizzed the girl about this, she quickly turned her face away from mine and mumbled something to the effect, 'We are not permitted to read the scan; you will have to see your doctor and he will explain it all to you.'

I took this to mean that she agreed with my prognosis, but didn't want to be the one to have to tell me.

How despondent I suddenly became. I thought, 'Oh God, I can deal with the one cancer I know I have, but, if there are more, then the picture is worse.'

I called my sister in Kennebunk and she, in an hour or so, came for me. I did not dare to tell her of my fears, when I tried to, I choked up to the extent that I couldn't continue. I wished that my wife June were there, and that she could be with me until I could find out the terrible news the next day, when I might see my doctor.

Needless to say, I did not sleep well that night. Imagine my joy, when arriving at the treatment center this morning to find June already there!

With great misgiving I requested to see my doctor after my treatment, and, with June present, told him I was prepared to hear the news of the bone scan. Dr. Gilbert went to the records, pulled my chart, opened it to a page and, holding it up for us both to see, said, 'Read this.' I put on my glasses, and read, 'Mr. Hopkins' bone scan is absolutely normal. There is no cancer in his body other than the known carcinoma in his chest!' Wow! Can you appreciate the significance of this!!! My lymph nodes in my chest show carcinoma. Once in the lymph nodes, it usually travels fast throughout the body. In me, it HAS NOT! Dear God! Thank you for small favors!"

(*Better than Dying* by William Hopkins,Hopkins Publications, pp.58-9)

Bill never mentioned his concern and the resulting anguish to me at the time. Had I known, I would have reassured him that the black spot that he saw in his pelvis was normal concentration of the radioactive material in the bladder. This is an unfortunate, painful experience that many of our patients go through. Unlike Mr. Hopkins, many others don't find out the results the next day; they have to wait, and suffer, for days or even weeks before they see the doctor.

Celina Schreiber, a good friend of my family, went for a mammogram at a Boston hospital. Following the procedure the radiologist told her that he was concerned about a spot on her mammogram and suggested further evaluation with a MRI. She went to the front desk to make that appointment and was told that the next available MRI was in two and a half months. Celina started to complain but was afraid she would lose her composure and left. That evening she spoke to my wife and I got on the line and joined the discussion. I asked her if I could make a call the next day and she gave her permission. The following morning I called the chief of radiology at the hospital and told her of our friend's experience. After I mentioned the two and a half month wait, I said nothing else. There was a slight gasp on the other end, then after a few seconds she said that I guess we have a problem. She asked me for the patient's name and said she would take care of it. I shudder to think how often I and other doctors order a test, like a bone or brain scan looking for a possible cause of symptoms and am not aware that there is a longer wait then is acceptable.

The art of communicating effectively with a patient and their family is a never ending process that is greatly dependent upon their feedback. I was treating a lady for lung cancer. She complained of a headache and I ordered a brain scan suspecting that she may have brain metastases. The following day I saw her and was pleased to report that her brain scan was negative. The next day she returned for her daily treatment and stopped me in the hall. She was not happy and said that she was so upset with me that she could not sleep because I said she had no brains when I told her that her brain scan was negative. I apologized for the misunderstanding and told her that when we do tests to evaluate for tumor involvement we report it as negative for tumor or positive. From that day on, I have reported the results of tests as either normal or abnormal. This lady reminded me that patients hang on every word a physician says and the wrong words can cause great concern and anguish.

How patients with lung cancer, who were referred to Maine Med for evaluation and treatment, were managed prior to the new protocol caused many sleepless nights for the patient and their family. A typical patient would go to his primary care physician with a cough and chest discomfort. A chest x-ray that day showed a mass in the lung and a CT scan two days later confirmed the mass and suggested enlarged nodes in the mediastinum. He was then referred to a pulmonologist for evaluation. The following week the pulmonologist saw the patient and ordered a bronchoscopy. This was done and he then returned to the pulmonologist several days after the procedure to discuss the pathological findings. The diagnosis of cancer was confirmed and the patient was then scheduled to see a chest surgeon. After the consultation, the surgeon arranged for a mediastinoscopy to evaluate the nodes in the chest and to determine if the patient was a candidate for surgical resection. After the surgical procedure he returned to the surgeon's office to discuss the pathological findings. If the patient was a surgical candidate, then the surgery was performed and if the tumor was inoperable, then the radiation and medical oncologists were consulted. Unfortunately the time it took from referral to the beginning of treatment could be two to three months and a repeat CT scan was often indicated to see how the tumor had changed.

How we evaluate patients has changed for the better. In the past it has been delivered at the schedule and convenience of the hospital and the doctors. It has transitioned to delivering health care centered on the needs of the patient. During the last decade Maine Med and many other hospitals have introduced a Nurse Navigator protocol where the patient is referred to the Navigator by the outside physician and he or she follows the patient and co-ordinates work-ups and consultations so that the entire process can occur in two to three weeks. That is patient centered care and the motto for Maine Med is now "Centered Around You".

GOD AND CANCER

Nothing rocks our foundation more than a diagnosis of cancer. Religion and our thought of God and the hereafter often take a back seat in our everyday lives until a life threatening event occurs.

I was raised in a Jewish section of Brooklyn where first and second generation American Jews where very respectful of their traditions. When I started Hebrew School I worried that if I entered the synagogue without wearing my skull cap I would be struck down by a lightning bolt. I was taught that if I led a good life and was respectful of the laws of our traditions, then I would be rewarded with good health and good fortune by the all-powerful, all seeing God. As I grew up I struggled with this concept, as I began to ponder the fate of the Jews during the Holocaust.

When I began my professional career in oncology I was confronted by many patients who felt that they were being punished for their previous sins. They wanted to know what they did to deserve this fate. A forty year old patient who died of a pelvic tumor gave me a book by Rabbi Harold Kushner titled *When Bad Things Happen to Good People*. She wrote inside the front cover that "This book changes nothing, but it makes much of my experience easier. I hope it has something for you too." I have read the book several times and I have often quoted it to bring comfort and acceptance to my patients. Kushner gives an example of the guilt people endure by telling of a couple whose only child, a nineteen year old woman, died suddenly during her freshman year at college. A blood vessel had burst in her brain while walking across the campus. Rabbi Kushner was called to console the parents. He walked into their home and the distraught mother said "You know, Rabbi, we didn't fast last Yom Kippur." Losing their only child was devastating enough but the thought that she died as a result of something they did was catastrophic.

Kushner wrote the book as a result of his own tragedy. His son was born with a rare genetic disease called progeria where the cells age abnormally fast. At age ten, his boy's hair turned gray and began falling out and his face wrinkled. He died of old age in his teens.

Kushner points out that bad things happen; planes crash, earthquakes kill thousands of people and tornados will destroy a row of houses and leave others untouched. God may have created the earth but does not control how things turn out. If God does not control who will live and who will die, then how does religion and God play a role? Patients who were not religious but whose families want them to become more spiritually involved to fight their disease often asked me what religion and prayer could do for them. Kushner answers this question in his book as follows. *"People who pray for miracles usually don't get miracles, any more than children who pray for bicycles, good grades, or boyfriends get them as a result of praying. But people who pray for courage, for strength to bear the unbearable, for the grace to remember what they have left instead of what they have lost, very often find their prayers answered. They discover that they have more strength, more courage than they ever knew themselves to have. Where did they get it? I would think that their prayers helped them find that strength. Their prayers helped them tap hidden reserves of faith and courage which were not available to them before."*

(*When Bad Things Happen To Good People* by Harold Kushner, Schocken Books, p.125)

When my patients asked me about the value of prayer I responded by relating an experience my son Scott had during his senior year in high school. He was working an evening shift at the Green Mountain Coffee Roasters in Monument Square. On a frigid winter evening, a large homeless man came in and sat down at a booth without ordering anything. Scott's manager, a petite woman in her early twenties asked Scott to accompany her as she was about to approach his table. Scott walked behind her and when she asked the man to leave he stood up threateningly and swore at her. Scott felt like running but the young woman stood her ground and so did Scott. A few moments later, he left. The manager told Scott that if he was not with her she never would have had the courage to stand her ground. "Although I walk through the shadow of death, I will fear no evil for thou art with me".

A minister with newly diagnosed rectal cancer came to see me. During our consultation I described what he had and how we were going to treat him. At the end of our discussion, which lasted over an hour, he said "You have told me what you are going to do but what can I do?" I answered that he could pray. He looked at me and nodded his head. Two months later I received a copy of a Southern Maine Christian newsletter containing an article by my patient with the headline "Dr. Gilbert said that I could pray". He then described how he was overwhelmed and distraught with his diagnosis and treatment and felt helpless. He needed his physician to remind him of the resources and strength he had in his faith and religion and what a comfort he found in it.

I treated a woman, who happened to be a nun, with post-hysterectomy irradiation for uterine cancer. She tolerated her treatments well and I followed her for the next three years. At that final visit she thanked me profusely for the care that she received and stated that she wished she could give me something to show her gratitude. I told her that I would greatly appreciate it if she would pray for me. A big smile and a tear came across her face and she assured me she would. For the next fifteen years, until her death, I received a Christmas card with a note that I was included in her daily prayers. Most times we think of what we should have said hours after the incident. My simple request said that I valued what she did and gave her the opportunity to give a very meaningful gift that was greatly appreciated.

Prayer and belief in God can provide courage and a purpose to not give up and a feeling that you are not alone. Prayer provides you and your loved ones with something that they and you can do to help. Many of my patients gained strength and encouragement from the thought that their friends had formed a prayer group or that their clergy had offered prayers on their behalf. Organized religion can provide a support system at times of need. Life cycle events, such as births, marriages, deaths and even illnesses have traditions and practices associated with them. The family and the community help celebrate happy occasions and comfort and assist during difficult times. In addition as one nears the end of life, if the belief is that you are going to a better place and will be reunited with long departed loved ones then that can bring comfort to the patient and their family.

Religion can also have a negative effect. Sometimes patients decide to forgo traditional medicine and depend on faith healing. When this comes up in my discussions with patients, I tell them that if I prayed rather than studied before my exams in medical school, I would not be their doctor today. God helps those who help themselves.

Many years ago I visited the Christian Science Pavilion at the Seattle World's Fair. I informed one of the practitioners in that pavilion that I was a medical student and had a question for her. I said that many people died of a Strep throat infection before the modern era of antibiotics. I asked her: if she had a Strep infection would she take Penicillin? She thought for several seconds and then responded that she could not honestly answer that question until she was actually confronted with it but that she would hope and pray to have the courage to not take it. If I had the opportunity to question her today, I would ask "if you ministered to a patient with a probable Strep throat, would you offer the information that Penicillin could be curative?"

RANDOM ACTS OF KINDNESS

Patients who are being treated for cancer are emotionally fragile and acts of support and kindness are especially appreciated at this vulnerable time.

A seventy year old lady was being treated for pancreatic carcinoma with radiotherapy and chemotherapy. That weekend, her children bought her a beautiful colorful flowered silk nightgown with a matching robe. She was an inpatient at MMC and was brought down for her treatment. While sitting in the waiting room she vomited all over her new outfit. She was distraught and crying. Bonnie McGarvey, our nurse, took her into an examining room and cleaned her up and gave her a hospital gown. She wrapped up her soiled nightgown and took it home where she washed and ironed it. The next day, when the patient came down for treatment, Bonnie took her into the examining room and changed her into her beautiful nightgown. The tears flowed as all saw her reaction of great appreciation. When I am sick and dying, I want somebody like Bonnie McGarvey to take care of me.

Another patient came in late for her treatment appointment in our Bath facility one cold winter morning and was very upset that she messed up the schedule. She told the other patients in the waiting room that it was so cold that morning that her arthritic hands could not put the car key into the ignition. The next day one of the patients asked to borrow her car for a few hours and had a remote starter installed so that by the time she was ready to leave her house, her car was warmed up. This random act of kindness affected all who witnessed it.

Gary Pike was a seventeen year old handsome, intelligent young man who was stricken with non-Hodgkin's lymphoma. His mother was very supportive and well informed about his illness and both she and Gary were appreciative of the care and caring that he received. After standard therapy the tumor progressed and he was scheduled for a bone marrow transplant in Boston as a last ditch effort to control his disease. I knew that he was a fan of car racing and I told him that if he received permission from his Boston doctors, I would take him to the Oxford 250, the biggest race in Maine. My friend, Mike Liberty, who then owned Oxford Speedway, told me that we could have a skybox to ourselves since there was one available that was not rented.

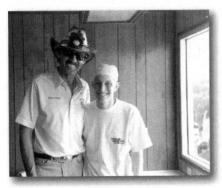

GARY PIKE AND RICHARD PETTY

We needed a separate space like a skybox since after bone marrow transplant one's immune defenses are low and one cannot be exposed to a large crowd. Gary came through his bone marrow transplant well and received permission to attend the race. The day of the race, Gary, his mother Trudy and I had the skybox to ourselves. The Grand Marshall for that year was Richard Petty, one of the greatest NASCAR racers of all time. He started the race and then came up to the skyboxes. He came into our box and stayed for almost forty-five minutes. He could not have been more friendly, caring and attentive to Gary. Gary had a big smile on his face as he posed with Richard for several pictures that his mother took. Gary asked him if he was concerned about getting hurt and he said that you take all the safety precautions, such as seat belts, helmets, and steel protective beams and then try not to think about the danger. He added that to be successful you must take chances and hopefully with some skill and a lot of good luck, it will work out. During that long visit I wondered how many hundreds of fans were waiting to speak to this famous man. Unfortunately the tumor recurred and Gary passed away several months later. His mother told me that on his bed post was the picture of Richard Petty and Gary that appears in this book.

Although I'm not a NASCAR fan, certainly the name of Richard Petty looms large across the world of celebrity. Today, our culture of hero worship builds both egos and bank accounts, but there are few opportunities to see the altruistic hero unless a camera or microphone is nearby. Richard Petty lived up to his nickname, 'King Richard' with a kindness and caring that made an incredible difference in the life of this young man. The 'Make A Wish' organization has offered their support through opportunities like this and the wisdom of that has played out in the lives of countless cancer patients.

Gary's mother told me that 'Make a Wish' did grant him a wish. Before he was diagnosed he won a music scholarship to Florida State University but was unable to attend because of his illness. His wish was to attend a FSU football game. They flew him and his folks down to Florida. They visited Disney World one day and then attended the FSU football game against the University of Florida at Gainesville. There were seventy thousand at the game and at halftime the loudspeaker announced that Gary was in the stands and invited him down to the field. There, surrounded by the cheerleaders, the band played a song for him and the cheerleaders displayed a huge sign which said that "FSU loves Gary Pike".

Following his death, his mother Trudi wanted to do something meaningful to remember Gary. She recalled the long lonely nights that she spent in a Boston hotel while he was fighting for his life in the hospital. Her husband joined her when he could but she had many meals and evenings by herself. In addition, the cost of staying at a Boston hotel was significant. As he was dying, Gary asked his mother to establish a hospitality home for families of patients hospitalized in the Portland area. Trudi and her friends established *Gary's House* in Portland in his memory which is a home away from home for the families of patients who are being cared for in the Portland hospitals. The camaraderie and support that these families give to each other is something that Trudi did not have when she was in Boston. She took her experience and made it a little easier, a little more comfortable and a little less stressful for those walking down the road behind her. Money was raised to renovate a Federal-style duplex with nine bedrooms and six community rooms on State Street in Portland and funds have been provided each year since to keep the facility functioning.

These three patients' lives were affected by cancer and at a low point for each of them, someone stepped in to pick up their spirit and make their ordeal more bearable. In doing so they made their own lives better. Kindness begets kindness.

SMOKING

My involvement with the American Cancer Society (ACS), as head of the Professional Education Committee and eventually President of the local chapter provided me with an opportunity to get the word out with regard to the negative effects of smoking. During this time I spoke at schools, community clubs and to cessation classes sponsored by the University of Southern Maine. One day I received a call from a local radio reporter, Don Huff, who subsequently moved on to WBZ in Boston but was working for WGAN at the time. He planned to do a five part series that was going to be aired during the week of the ACS annual Great American Smoke out and wanted to also speak to a patient for one of the segments. For most of the interview I reviewed the devastating health effects of smoking and how cessation of smoking could be very beneficial. Then I introduced him to a forty-two year old former smoker who was in the hospital being treated for her lung cancer with brain metastases. My patient talked about how she started to smoke in high school because it was the cool thing to do and that it was a pleasurable habit that was hard to break. Toward the end of the interview she looked directly at Don Huff and said, "The worst thing about my diagnosis is the terrible guilt feeling I have every time I look into my nine year old baby's eyes and realize that because of my weakness and selfishness, he will have to grow up without his mother". There was a stunned silence in the room. The broadcast featuring the patient's comment received the award for the best interview in the State that year.

A very bright and interested group of high school students from Boothbay Harbor came to our Department at MMC for a discussion on radiation therapy and the consequences of smoking. During our talk, a girl in the back of the room said, "Doc, I will give you the cause and effect of smoking and lung cancer but I don't buy the relationship of smoking and heart disease". I asked the thirty-five students how many knew of someone who died suddenly from a heart attack when they were in their forties, fifties or early sixties and never made it to the hospital. Eleven hands went up. Then I asked them how many of those eleven were nonsmokers. No hands were raised. I looked at the girl and she said that she was convinced. The ratio of smokers to non-smokers for sudden death is eleven to one for people under the age of sixty-five.

That question concerning sudden death became part of my smoking presentation. A year later I spoke to about two hundred and fifty Navy men and women at Brunswick Naval Air Station as part of a health symposium featuring the importance of smoking cessation. I asked the question to the audience about sudden death below the age of mid-sixties and fifty hands went up. I then asked how many of those fifty did not smoke. One hand went up and he said he was not sure if his relative smoked or not.

During my lectures to the smoking cessation classes at USM, I cited a study done in the 1950's in England. All of the new births in the county over a month were registered and the mothers filled out an extensive questionnaire. They asked for general health status, education level, living conditions, if they smoked and so on. Records from the school system were obtained when these children were seven and eleven years of age. They had information on height, weight and IQ. They found that there was a statistically significant decrease in all three in the children whose mothers smoked during pregnancy. I said that I did not feel that these findings were all related to smoking during pregnancy but rather to continued exposure to second hand smoke during their childhood. I asked my class how they felt about a study where some infants and young children would be placed in a closed room where smoke was introduced. My students were appalled at the thought of this. I told them they should think about that the next time they drive by a car on a cold day with children sitting in the backseat and a parent smoking in the front. I am very proud that the State of Maine passed a law that outlaws smoking even in one's own car, if children under the age of sixteen are present.

ASBESTOS LITIGATION

C aring for patients sometimes requires getting involved in matters that they do not teach in medical school.

Several years ago Peter Rubin asked me to review some cases as an expert witness in the asbestos litigation trials. He was the chief defense counsel for certain asbestos companies and asked me to testify about the relation-ship of smoking and lung cancer. Asbestos was effective in preventing fires and was used extensively to insulate pipes on Navy ships during WW II and in the fifties and sixties. Unfortunately asbestos fibers float in the air and if inhaled by the workers could cause scarring of the lung and its out-er covering, called the pleura, producing asbestosis. Exposure to asbestos increased the risk of developing lung cancer and was the major cause of mesothelioma, a malignant tumor of the pleura.

The litigation process in the U.S. is important since it provides a mecha-nism for injured parties to receive compensation when they are wrongfully harmed and punishes the offending party to pay that compensation as well as pay the lawyers who make the system work. With asbestos and ship-building it becomes more complicated. The U.S. government, which pro-vided the specifications for the required products, cannot be sued except in rare situations. The shipyard, where the work was done, is usually not considered liable. The asbestos manufacturers, however, who produced a product that was requested during WW II and in the Cold War, can be held accountable even though that product fit all requested specifications. In addition, the executives of the asbestos companies who were in charge twenty to sixty years ago are long gone. The defendants are mainly compa-nies who used to supply asbestos products and now thousands of employees and stockholders of those companies must bear the costs for the damages.

There were hundreds of potential plaintiffs; each one entitled to their own depositions, trial with a jury and expert witnesses. In Maine, our distinguished federal judge, Judge Edward Gignoux tried to streamline the asbestos docket by combining ten or so plaintiffs into one jury trial. I should digress and inform the reader that Judge Gignoux received national attention when he was asked to go to Chicago and retry the Chicago Seven after their mistrial with Judge Hoffman. He was given the Jurist of the Year award for that trial by the American Bar Association. In Florida he tried Judge Alcee Hastings, then a Federal Judge for accepting a bribe but was acquitted when his alleged co-conspirator refused to testify. Hastings was impeached and convicted by Congress in 1989 and became the sixth Federal Judge to be removed from office. After he was removed from the bench he ran for Congress and has been there since 1993. What does that tell you about our legislature!

I enjoyed the intellectual challenge of being an expert witness. In one trial with ten plaintiffs, I was listed as an expert witness for the defense in seven cases for those who smoked and developed lung cancer, and was listed as a plaintiff's expert witness for a patient of mine with mesothelioma. My patient's lawyer did not call me to testify at the trial since that would have provided me more credibility for my previous testimony for the defense. My favorite interchange at trial was with a well-known Pittsburgh lawyer who asked me if I was an epidemiologist and if not, how I can be so sure that there was a relationship between smoking and lung cancer. I answered that each year our Department saw about two hundred new patients with lung cancer and 97% were either smokers or ex-smokers while only 30% of the U.S. adult population smoked, so I did not need an epidemiologist to tell me there was a causal relationship. The lawyer immediately backed off and went on to another question.

I was turned off with the litigation process by two experiences. The first was my sixty-three years old patient who was dying from mesothelioma and was being treated with radiotherapy for chest wall pain. At our last follow-up visit, about three weeks before he died, he told me that he had dropped his lawsuit against the asbestos companies. I told him and his wife that I was very disappointed since mesothelioma cases were the first in line to deserve compensation. He explained that they had settled with several asbestos companies but had not received any money to date. He asked his lawyer where the money was and he replied that the lawyer received 40%, legal costs were an additional 3% and the remaining 57% had liens by Anthem Blue Cross and Workman's Compensation for their expenditures during his illness. He then asked his lawyer what the bottom line was and the lawyer told him that they would probably get $350,000 and the patient's share would be approximately $50,000. He told the lawyer that he was going to drop the case since he did not want to go to all this trouble just to make others rich. The lawyer responded that even if he dropped his case, Blue Cross and Workman's Comp would hire him to receive their compensation. I encouraged him to continue the case for the good of his family. He answered that before a deposition he gets so nervous that he cannot sleep for a whole week. His wife tearfully added that she did not want that money and would prefer that he was not hassled in his current state.

This session really upset me. I never realized that the lawyer's percentage came off the top and the insurance companies would have a lien only on the plaintiff's settlement. The total cost to the asbestos companies, including the settlement and the costs of defending the suit would cost close to $500,000. The victim, who was suffering a painful, premature death, would get 10%. The lawyers involved had many similar cases while this was the only chance for the victim to provide for his widow. That evening I called a trusted friend, the late Judge Sidney Wernick who was a retired Justice of the Maine Supreme Court. He listened to my story and suggested that I call the wife and ask her to contact the involved judge or the Bar Association and they would immediately strike the 40% to 33%, which is not a lot of money but would increase my patient's total by almost 50%. In my patient's case, of the $350,000 settlement the lawyer would normally get 33% or about $117,000. The legal fees would be 3% or $10,500, the insurance companies would be reimbursed $148,000 and the plaintiff's widow would get only $74,500.

A couple of years later I brought up this case with the actual plaintiff's lawyer when he came to my office to discuss another patient. I asked him, professional to professional, if there wasn't a better way to handle these cases. He did not respond. Several years later I discussed the case with Judge Gignoux, who officiated at the trial. He listened and sadly shook his head and said the system is not perfect, but it is the best we have.

The other major turn off to the litigation process was a deposition I gave on a Thursday afternoon on January 12, when a freezing rain was falling in Portland. I remember the date since the plaintiff's lawyer flew up from the South and being superstitious, would not fly home on Friday the 13th. The last plane out of Portland to get him home, left at 6 P.M. The deposition concerned a man with lung cancer who smoked heavily for several years. I had previously given at least three depositions and court testimony in similar cases and all the involved lawyers had the transcripts of that testimony. Peter Rubin received calls from lawyers from Boston, New Hampshire and Providence asking if the deposition would be re-scheduled due to the freezing rain. Since the plaintiff's lawyer was already in Portland, the deposition would proceed as planned. To my amazement, at least twelve lawyers were present, the plaintiff's lawyer being the only one to ask me questions. All the other lawyers represented the different asbestos companies and all with their meters running for a case that was settled out of court the following week. When I calculated the cost of that deposition I realized how wasteful and very inefficient the process is, except for the lawyers.

If the real goal of tort litigation is to compensate the victim, then we cannot be satisfied paying 10% to 20% of the total cost to the injured party. For cases like asbestos, we should have a high level trial. The scientific data should be presented to a qualified group of scientists who objectively evaluate the expert witness data. Then a panel can allocate fair compensation for different situations, such as mesothelioma, lung cancer in a non-smoker, compared to a lung cancer patient with a heavy smoking history. A similar type of allocation system was set up following the World Trade Center attack. This system would not work as well for the lawyers involved, but of course, they are not the victims.

I have great respect and admiration for the legal profession. Lawyers who take on a new problem and have to research the facts and the precedents and then build a case deserve to get 33%, especially if they are not guaranteed compensation if they lose in court. However, asbestos is another story. It has been tried hundreds of times and all of the steps are laid out in books. The settlement is practically assured so that the lawyer has little risk for not being compensated. Unlike the lawyer who has many such cases, the victim has only one chance to collect and provide for his family. For the lawyer to receive 33% from the top from many clients while doing work a paralegal could do isn't justice, in my opinion. The fact that the legal system does not address this injustice and protect the victim is a sad commentary. A proposed Federal law called the 'Fair Act' would address this injustice but the lobbyists for the Trial Lawyers have effectively killed it. Thus the plaintiff attorneys will continue to receive one third of the billions of dollars set aside to compensate the asbestos victims. All those who are paid to provide justice for the citizens including the Federal and State Legislatures, lawyers, the judges and the Attorney General in Washington, share responsibility for this travesty.

YOU HAVE TO LAUGH

"EVERY TIME YOU FIND SOME HUMOR IN A DIFFICULT SITUATION, YOU WIN."
                                        SUE FITZMAURICE

"I GOT THE BILL FOR MY SURGERY. NOW I KNOW WHY THOSE DOCTORS WERE WEARING MASKS."
                                        JAMES H. BOREN

I was treating a woman in her young forties for breast cancer. For many years she had been very leery of chemicals and additives in her food and in various products. For her to be receiving radiation therapy and chemotherapy, with these poisons circulating throughout her body, was a traumatic experience. She was in the middle of a six week course of irradiation to her breast after a lumpectomy. One day she stormed into the Bath facility and confronted me by saying "You of all people, how can you allow them to spray those cancer causing chemicals on your lawn?" Since we had a good relationship I thought for a second and responded, "It's good for business". She held her breath for several seconds and then burst out laughing.

A seventy-one year old man returned for a check-up to our department a few months after completing his course of radiotherapy to his prostate. While standing next to our nurse's station, he told my nurse and me that his urologist gave him samples for Cialis to treat his erectile dysfunction. As he was leaving the urologist's office he went up to the nurse and said, "Let me get this straight. If my erection lasts longer than three hours I am supposed to call you?" She said, "Oh yes, by all means!" and we all shared a good laugh.

I was doing a rectal exam on a man with prostate cancer. As I was probing he asked, "What are you doing, drilling for oil?" I answered that I never get oil but sometimes I get gas.

During my radiology residency I did an angiogram on a sixteen year old girl. She was very anxious and I gave her some Valium prior to the procedure. At the end of the exam I asked her how she handled it. She looked up at me, gave me a big smile and with a slight slurring of her speech asked, "Can I come back for another angiogram tomorrow?"

Too Close For Comfort

As an oncologist I was reminded on a daily basis of how fortunate I was to have my family's good health. However, none of us walks through life untouched and my response to cancer when it arrived on my doorstep made me personally more attached and more empathetic with my patients.

My father died from colon cancer. It was located in the sigmoid portion of the colon and was resected cleanly. He did well without adjuvant treatment for five years and then developed a cough. X-rays revealed a mass in the right lung and biopsy revealed that this was a metastasis from the colon. He received local irradiation and chemo in Florida and had a good quality of life for another four years, before he lost his battle with cancer when the tumor spread to his pericardium. He was seventy-three years old.

Following my father's recurrence but while he was still alive, I consulted on a man in his seventies with metastatic colon cancer. It had spread to his lower thoracic vertebra and was threatening his spinal cord, which could cause paralysis in his legs. That evening I began to worry that my father could have painful symptoms, like my patient and felt it would be too uncomfortable for me to treat this man. I actually considered but did not act on having one of my colleagues take over his management. As it turned out, we were able to alleviate my patient's discomfort and my father never ended up developing any painful metastases.

My niece Elise was a beautiful, lively, new mother at the age of thirty-four when she developed a very aggressive mediastinal lymphoma. I learned that this was a sub-type of lymphoma that occurs mainly in women in their thirties and is often associated with pregnancy. That however may coincidently be related to the age group. It was a type with a higher mortality rate than other lymphomas in spite of aggressive treatment. Although she lived in Florida I arranged for a friend of mine who is one of the leading physicians treating lymphoma, to evaluate and treat her at the Dana Farber

Cancer Center in Boston. Her parents and family members provided her with a wonderful blanket of support when she came to Boston. However, despite having only transient responses to the best treatment that was then available, Elise passed away two years later. The loss was devastating and emphasized to me the limitations of what medicine can accomplish.

About five years later I consulted on a thirty-three year old woman who was diagnosed when her first child was two months old with the same aggressive mediastinal lymphoma as my niece. She came to our initial consultation with her baby and her Mom. When I looked at her all I could see was Elise and I feared that she would have the same fate. Again, I considered having another physician manage her treatment; however I was the only doctor at the Bath facility. She was treated with four months of chemo and she had a good partial response followed by five weeks of consolidation radiotherapy to the area of gross disease. She tolerated all of her treatment very well and I followed her carefully. After three years with no evidence of recurrence, I told her about my niece and how hard it was for me to treat her. We had a very emotional discussion and she told me how much she appreciated the difficulty of my situation and how grateful she was to have survived. Several weeks later she sent the following note:

Dear Dr. Gilbert,

Thank you for being such a vital part of my survival team! I truly appreciate and could sense the care and concern you gave me and I'm so thankful that you shared your side of the story with me. In the gentlest way you always made the reality of my health clear and at the same time gave me hope that I could beat it. I hope I can pass along some of the same kindness and support. I will hold your niece and family dear, they have offered great inspiration.

My best to you always,

My third experience with cancer concerning a family member was when my wife was diagnosed. Carol had a lump on the sole of her left foot for many years, which we had dismissed as being the result of a splinter that had become imbedded and callused over. It had been there for so long that she said "If it was malignant, I would be dead by now" and continued to ignore it. Over time she began to limp more and had difficulty walking long distances, and finally she decided to see an orthopedic surgeon who specialized in foot surgery. He felt it was a benign fibroma and scheduled an out-patient surgical procedure. The operation went well and the surgeon said that the tumor was easily removed.

The following Monday I was in the middle of a busy clinic when I received a call from the pathologist at Mercy Hospital. I had called his office a couple of days before and asked him to review a path report on a patient of mine and check on the adequacy of the margin around the tumor. He told me that he was not calling about my patient but about my wife. He said that he completed his analysis of Carol's operative specimen and he thought it was a malignant Epithelioid Schwannoma and the margin of resection did not seem to be adequate. These tumors often start as benign and then have malignant degeneration. They are an unusual lesion of a peripheral nerve sheath and need to be removed. There is a significant chance that the tumor can recur locally if the resection margin is not adequate.

Needless to say, I was stunned. I thanked the pathologist and went to my office to take a couple of breaths. I decided to call my mentor at the Mass General, Dr. Herman Suit who was widely recognized as a leading expert on the radiotherapy of soft tissue sarcoma. However, first I had to get through my morning clinic and see my four remaining patients. Fortunately they were follow-up visits and all were doing well.

When I finished seeing my last patient I went to my office and called Dr. Suit. I told him that this was a phone call I never wanted to make to him. I told him of Carol's lump and the resulting pathology report. Initially he was quiet and then said that he had to make arrangements with a few key people and would call me back in a few minutes. Twenty minutes later he called to say that he arranged to have Dr. Dempsey Springfield, a top orthopedic surgeon, consult with us at 10 A.M. on Wednesday. During that visit the slides would be reviewed by the pathologist who specialized in sarcoma. Dr. Suit also scheduled a MRI of the foot at that time. He did ask that she get a chest CT scan at Maine Med prior to the appointment. Dr. Suit had a special close relationship with many of his residents and fellows and treated us as if we were part of his family.

Carol had her chest CT scan the next day and when I reviewed it with the radiologist, he noted a small nubbin of tissue in the lung, probably an old scar from a viral pneumonia but he could not rule out a small tumor. He advised a follow-up scan in four to six months. The next day we went to Boston with the scans and pathology specimen and were greeted by a very concerned Dr. Suit. He led us to Dr. Springfield's office where he stayed with us for the consultation. They went down to pathology to review the slides with the pathologist and returned to talk to us. Dr. Springfield said that the tumor was definitely malignant with margin involvement and his plan was to get adequate margins by removing the second toe with its meta-tarsal with the result hopefully being a fully functional foot. He told us that the surgery would be challenging since he had to protect the blood vessels and the adjacent nerves to prevent damage to the adjacent tissue. He added that if this operation did not get clear margins, the next procedure would most likely be a below the knee amputation to give the most useful function of the leg. He scheduled the surgery for the following Tuesday.

I had previously scheduled a three day cruise out of Miami that Friday to celebrate Carol's fiftieth birthday, which was the following week. We decided not to cancel; a good diversion was the best defense that weekend. We called our children, Scott and Alison and told them that Mom needed further surgery for a low grade malignant tumor in her foot and she was going to be operated on the following week. Scott was at medical school in St. Louis and Alison was in the Peace Corps in Costa Rica. I informed them that we were going on the cruise that weekend and I would call after the surgery was over. We decided not to tell anybody else since we were going to be out of town for the time up to the surgery. The cruise proved to be a godsend. Rather than sit home and think all weekend we were kept busy enjoying the sunshine, activities and plenty of delicious food.

The surgery went well and the pathology report described that the margin was three millimeters clear from the tumor. Was this few millimeters adequate or should she receive post-operative radiotherapy? This is a decision I would usually be asked to make on a weekly basis. The foot is exposed to significant trauma and does not do as well as other tissue after irradiation. Fortunately, I left the decision up to Dr. Suit who said that we would follow it closely and not give radiotherapy at this time.

The surgery was successful and the tumor never returned. Carol has had full use of her foot and has golfed, skied and walked with only minor effects from the procedure. The follow-up CT of the chest showed no change and that density was considered to be scar tissue.

This personal experience with cancer from the family's view point taught me some great lessons. I was very relieved to be in Dr. Suit's able hands and allow him to make all of the major decisions concerning Carol's treatment. The anxiety and pressure of dealing with this diagnosis without worrying about second guessing myself was a huge relief. In this book I have repeatedly stressed that the doctor is a guide and the patient should be given the information they need to make their own decisions. I am grateful that Dr. Suit didn't ask us how we wanted to proceed.

We returned to Dr. Springfield's office six weeks after surgery and while sitting in the waiting room a man close to my age, entered pushing his wife in a wheelchair. She was thin, very pale and had lost her hair. I gasped to myself and felt queasy. I realized how close we had come to having the same situation as that unfortunate couple. It occurred to me that as an oncologist who navigates these scenarios on a daily basis, my reactions and emotions weren't far removed from what my patients all experience. It gave me a greater appreciation for a lay person's reaction to the same situation.

WILL TO LIVE

"BAD THINGS DO HAPPEN; HOW I RESPOND TO
THEM DEFINES MY CHARACTER AND THE QUALITY
OF MY LIFE. I CAN CHOOSE TO SIT IN PERPETUAL
SADNESS, IMMOBILIZED BY THE GRAVITY OF MY
LOSS, OR I CAN CHOOSE TO RISE FROM THE PAIN
AND TREASURE THE MOST PRECIOUS GIFT I HAVE
— LIFE ITSELF."   WALTER ANDERSON

Patients who have metastatic, incurable cancer tend to do better if
they have a purpose for living such as a wedding to attend or a family
event.

I cared for a patient who was dying from a cancer at the base of his tongue.
After having had surgery, high dose radiotherapy and chemo the tumor was
recurring. He was in some pain, had difficulty swallowing and was losing
weight when I saw him during a follow-up visit. He had appropriate pain
medicine but he assured me that I should not worry about him because he
was not going to allow the tumor to progress much further. He had plans to
end his life before the discomfort became intolerable and he was unable to
swallow. We had a long discussion and I gave him an appointment to return
in six weeks, not expecting to see him again. Six weeks later he showed up
having gained ten pounds. He gave me a smile when I showed my pleasure
and surprise at how well he looked. He told me that a funny thing happened on the way to the cemetery; his wife had a positive mammogram
and needed treatment for her breast cancer. He now had a mission and a
purpose to continue. The patient took care of himself and his wife until her
treatment was completed and then passed away two months later.

A friend of mine was in her forties when she was diagnosed with breast
cancer. It had metastasized to her bones when the youngest of her three

children, a daughter, was in the eighth grade. The patient looked me straight in the eye and said she had a responsibility to raise that girl to adulthood and she was not going anywhere until she went to college. Fortunately she responded to systemic and local treatment and died five years later during Christmas vacation of her daughter's freshman year in college.

Another patient was failing with bone metastases from prostate cancer. Although I was able to control his pain with local irradiation and pain meds, he began to question if it was all worth the trouble. I asked him what would give him pleasure and he said he would like to spend more time with his grown children and grandkids. I discussed with him a plan to have each of his children schedule a visit. This gave him an opportunity to spend quality time with each one and gave him a purpose for the last months of his life. The most meaningful compliments are the ones you hear via a third party. My neighbor attended my patient's funeral and told me that during his son's eulogy, he said that "Dr. Gilbert could not have cared more for his own father then he did for mine".

Don't Give Up Too Soon

I have learned over the years that if a patient who is in reasonable shape presents with what appears to be an advanced, incurable tumor, a trial of chemotherapy with or without radiotherapy is indicated. There is no way to know whether or not that patient will have a significant response to treatment without trying. If the tumor responds and the patient tolerates the treatment, then we can proceed with additional therapy.

This approach proved to be a good decision for a seventy-one year old lady who called herself 'the miracle patient'. She presented with a locally advanced cervical cancer that had invaded both pelvic sidewalls, partially obstructing both ureters (the tubes that connect the kidneys to the bladder) and the rectum. Our gynecological oncologist, Charlie Boyce decided to be aggressive with her and planned to divert the ureters and bowel so that she could be treated better with radiation therapy and chemotherapy. At surgery he found a huge pelvic mass that was fixed to the pelvic sidewalls and some enlarged para-aortic lymph nodes (draining nodes in the mid and upper abdomen). He decided to abort his operation and referred her back to us for palliative treatment. We started off with chemo alone and the patient had an excellent partial response with reduced ureteral and bowel obstruction. Since that worked we proceeded with pelvic irradiation and concomitant chemo. She responded to that treatment and then received an intra-cavitary radioactive implant in the vagina and uterus and an external radiotherapy boost to the pelvic sidewalls. With no definite residual tumor in the pelvis, we gave her a course of radiotherapy to the para-aortic nodes. She did well. Eight years later she developed a colon cancer in the hepatic flexure, high in the abdomen and far from our irradiated portal. At the time of surgical resection of the colon cancer, no residual tumor was found from the previous malignancy in the pelvis and she died fifteen years after her initial therapy, with no evidence of cancer.

One of my patients who proved to me the importance of perseverance was a fifty year old man with renal cell cancer. I was treating him for a recurrence in the area of the duodenum, after his right kidney was removed. I gave him palliative radiotherapy which stopped his upper GI bleeding for only a few weeks. The patient was sent to Boston where the surgeon did a palliative Whipple procedure to remove the head of the pancreas and the duodenum. I thought that was aggressive surgery for a man with incurable disease; however he tolerated the surgery and was able to enjoy a good quality of life. Over the next eight years he had multiple resections of metastatic deposits in the liver, lung and soft tissue and I was amazed by the results his surgical team was able to achieve. Fortunately for him, renal cell cancer is one of those tumors that can progress slowly.

Sally was sixty-five years old when she presented with an unusual and challenging tumor. She was diagnosed with a cholangiocarcinoma. This is a malignant tumor of the bile ducts that is often diagnosed after it has spread and very difficult to cure. She had mild jaundice and was found to have an enlarged bile duct and a blood marker, Ca19-9 of over 3,000 (normal should be less than 37). This is a tumor associated antigen that is most often associated with cancer of the pancreas and the bile ducts. Sally was told that this was extensive enough to be incurable and she accepted it. The medical oncologist and I treated her with a conservative regimen of 5-FU chemotherapy and concomitant radiotherapy delivering 4500 cGy to the hepatic hilum, the area where a lump and dilated bile ducts were seen on CT scan. She tolerated the combined chemo/RT well and I ordered a repeat CT scan and Ca19-9 blood test prior to her return for a follow-up visit one month later. The lump on CT had shrunk and her Ca19-9 was down to 30, which is within normal range. I did not expect this remarkable response and I asked her to come in for a discussion with her husband. I went over the scans and the blood marker results and I recommended that she have an exploration of the abdomen to assess the status of the residual tumor and the possibility that it could be resected. At first she refused and said that she accepted her fate and that she did not want to go through a great deal of tests and procedures trying to prevent the inevitable. She and her husband finally agreed to be seen by a surgeon for a second opinion. She underwent a laparotomy and the surgeon resected the extra-hepatic ducts. This included the area where the lump was seen on the initial CT scan. The pathology was reported as scar tissue with no viable tumor cells detected. She called me from her hospital bed and thanked me for my encouragement and for not giving up on her.

Sally did well for four years with no significant symptoms. However the Ca 19-9 marker started to creep up to about 100. A repeat CT revealed some small lesions in the right lobe of the liver and it was concluded that the tumor was involving the right biliary ducts. She underwent surgery that removed the right lobe of her liver which contained the remaining tumor. It has been eleven years since her partial hepatectomy and there is no evidence of disease. Recently Carol and I were honored to attend Sally's and her husband Bill's eightieth birthday party with their extended family. They are both doing very well. The initial treatment she received was low dose and not aggressive and none of her doctors expected a dramatic result. When the tumor response exceeded our expectations, we adjusted our thinking and became more aggressive. She was very fortunate that the entire residual tumor was in the right lobe of the liver and it was amenable to complete resection.

The following is another case that taught me to not give up too early. This patient presented with extensive pancreatic cancer. She had surgery at the Lahey Clinic where they found a large tumor in the pancreas that spread to adjacent nodes and to the adjacent liver. They aborted the surgery after the biopsies came back as small cell carcinoma. This is an unusual cell type for the pancreas and is known to spread quickly but can be responsive to chemotherapy and irradiation. It is most commonly seen in the lung. Tom Ervin, a medical oncologist, and I discussed the case and decided to treat her with a protocol used for small cell carcinoma of the lung. We started her off with two cycles of chemotherapy and then a combined course of irradiation and chemo. She tolerated her treatments well and fortunately had a total response. She did not recur for the three years that I followed her.

I would not have given any of these patients much of a chance for controlling their tumors or for providing them with a good quality of life when they first presented. They did not have much hope of being cured but had excellent initial responses which encouraged their doctors to be more aggressive. When a young doctor asked me what I was going to do next, I would respond that the patient will always tell you what to do. If the tumor responds well and the patient tolerates treatment then you continue active treatment. These patients taught me that a physician does not have all the answers and should not give up pre-maturely. When I came to Maine I knew the data from the articles and textbooks and repeated it to my inquiring patients. It wasn't long before I realized that statistics were of little help when predicting how an individual patient will respond. In my later years when a patient asked me how much time he had left I would tell him that I used to think I knew the answer but now I know I don't.

END OF LIFE

One of the most important chapters of one's life is the final one.
After we die, our family and friends will long remember how we
handled our last days.

Unlike sudden death due to heart attack or stroke, cancer provides us
with an opportunity to tell our loved ones how much they mean to
us and to address important details such as economic issues. Families cope
better if they are prepared. In the U.S. more time, energy and financial resources are wasted trying to 'prevent the tide from coming in', rather than
to plan for and deal with the inevitability of dying. A significant percentage of Medicare costs are spent on the last couple of months of life partly
because patients and their families often regard death as a dirty word that
must be avoided at any cost. The absolute finality of death often compels
patients and their families to search for that life saving miracle, leaving no
stone unturned.

Physicians are not always helpful when they tell patients that if the current treatment does not work, then there is another one to try. If our goal
is for a patient to live forever, we will fail every time. A better objective
would be to enable him or her to die comfortably and with dignity. Unfortunately physicians get little if any training on how to do this important
work. Thinking back over a thirty-three year career, how I dealt with
cancer patients in the first decade compared to the latter third is the best
example of just how much my patients and their families taught me. I am
a better physician as a result. During my first decade of practice I did not
want any patient to die on my shift. I was so concerned that I would over-
look something that I kept on pushing, even beyond any reasonable hope
of success. After a few years of practice I realized that for every patient
with advanced disease that did well with aggressive treatment, there were

many more patients who had significant morbidity and eventual reduction in the length and quality of their lives as a result of continued oncologic treatment.

My management involving end of life cases was greatly affected by the following emotional experience, validating my belief that there is a time to treat and a time to let go. I had been taking care of Fran, a sixty-three year old lady with metastatic breast cancer for about eight years. She, her husband and her parents were longtime friends. She was failing with painful bone metastases and liver involvement and was admitted to the hospital for radiotherapy to a painful bone metastasis. On the day she was to start her short course of palliative treatment I received a frantic call from her daughter, Paula, who was at her mother's bedside. She told me that her mother was refusing to come down for treatment and she asked me to come up to speak to her. On my way into the room I reviewed her chart which showed significant deterioration of her liver function blood tests. Fran told me that she had fought hard but was now tired and did not have the strength to fight anymore. I told her that that was not unreasonable and that she was not making a mistake. I made eye contact with her daughter and there was a calm expression on her face. She understood my message and pulled up a chair next to the bed and sat down, holding her mom's hand. I believe that both Fran and Paula were entering into what Kubler Ross calls 'the acceptance stage'. Rather than frantically fighting off the tumor for the remainder of her life, mother and daughter spent her last two days together reminiscing, laughing, crying and talking for hours and Paula told me it was one of her most precious experiences. A few days after she died I received the following letter.

Dear Dr. Gilbert,

My mom was a great lady in many ways, and I know that her death will leave me with a sense of loss that can never be completely healed. That sense of loss, however, will always be held in balance by all of the things that she gave me and that I learned from her.

The greatest lesson that she taught me was to live life to its fullest because it is precious; to fight for as long as one can to live that life, and to let go when it is time. Thank you for helping her to fight and later for giving her permission to go. It seems to me that you are a unique physician. You were personally invested in healing my mother, but you seemed to understand that her very soul was central to the healing of her body. Once it was past the time for her body to repair itself, you gave great respect to her soul. I will be forever grateful for your simple words, "Fran, you are not making a mistake."

Thank you for taking care of my mother, and thank you for being so caring and respectful of Eric's and my needs. I hope that you are always blessed with the strength to continue with your work, because you are a gifted doctor and a wise man. I am sure that there must be some days when your work seems like the hardest thing in the world. Today, at least, I hope that you can know that you made a difference in my mom's life and therefore in the lives of her children.

Very truly yours,

Paula

I wrote the following note back to her.

Dear Paula,

Thank you for your beautiful note. As you mentioned, my work has wonderful highs when we assist a patient safely through the night-mare called cancer, but we also have terrible lows when confronted with the frustrations of realizing the limits of what we can achieve. To get through those lows, I often escape to those notes from pa-tients and families that remind me that we can affect others in a meaningful way.

Your letter is one of the most meaningful that I have ever received, not only for its content, but because your parents and grandparents mean, and meant, a lot to me. I will always treasure your letter and will re-read it on those occasions when I need a pick-me-up.

Please accept my sincere condolences. I can truly appreciate the enormity of your loss.

Yours truly,

Stu Gilbert

The experience and communication with Fran's daughter had a profound and lasting effect on me and how I practiced medicine. The importance of helping the patient fight her tumor was just as important as helping her reach the acceptance stage. I became more appreciative of the value of hospice and palliative care and became more focused on preparing my patients and their families for the time when aggressive treatment was counterproductive.

I recently had the pleasure to talk to her daughter and she wrote the following about how her mother's passing changed her life.

"Witnessing my mother's final six weeks of life was the most difficult thing I have ever done. I moved to Maine from New Jersey with my five month old baby Josh, leaving my three older kids with my husband. It was clear to me that as soon as she learned that her cancer had jumped to her liver, she shut down her desire to live. All her life she was sweet and uncomplicated and uncomplaining. But now at the end, she was mad. I learned that I couldn't shape her death for her. All I could give her was my presence. My presence was more than enough.

I felt very alone through those long weeks. Twenty years ago, I was a young mom and did not feel equipped to deal with so many hard decisions. If not for Dr. Gilbert and several amazing nurses at Maine Med, I am not sure that I could have made it through.

After my mom's death I realized that it was time for me to get on with my long held dream. After twelve years as a social worker, it was time to study for the rabbinate. If I could accompany my own mother on the path to her death, then I could do it for others. Before sheloshim (30 days of mourning) was over, I was in the office of the Dean of the Jewish Theological Seminary Rabbinical School, talking about entering his institution. Being a social worker had been satisfying and meaningful work. Becoming a rabbi meant that I could add the God-piece of the picture. In my years as a congregational rabbi, I have tried to make sure that no family member of a dying person would ever feel alone. I commit myself to patient, empathic accompanying, listening, witnessing -- in memory of my mother."

The following two patients illustrate end of life decisions. The first was a man in his sixties who was presented at a monthly tumor conference in a regional hospital that I attended on a regular basis. He was admitted the night before with an extensive lung cancer that was compressing his spinal cord. This is considered a radiotherapy emergency and they were looking to transfer the patient to Maine Med. On further inquiry I found that he also had partial tumor compression of the superior vena cava (the large vein that drains the upper half of the body), a large lung primary with metastases to the mediastinum, opposite lung, the liver and to the brain. He was very ill and barely coherent. At the conference I said that every once in a while a patient should be allowed to die without a $50,000 medical bill. The patient passed away within thirty-six hours.

The other was a man who was diagnosed with two incurable cancers; a small cell lung cancer that metastasized and acute leukemia. I saw him since he had brain metastases from his lung cancer. I explained to him that our goal was to treat the brain lesions, shrink them down so that he could have control of his body for the rest of his life. The patient grabbed my hand and told me he did not want to extend his life just to spend it in hospitals feeling sick. He asked if all this planned treatment would be worth it. I told him that I did not know; some patients respond well and have some quality of life while others became sicker and weaker with each treatment and have nothing to show for it. Six months later he returned to our department for palliative treatment to a painful bone lesion. He was lying on a stretcher in the hall and looked awful. I asked him if the past few months were worth taking the treatment and he answered promptly that it absolutely was. He passed away a couple of weeks later.

When a patient is informed that their tumor has spread to the bone or lung and that their cancer is no longer curable, many will have the initial response to throw in the towel and give up. Why prolong the agony with chemo and radiotherapy and enduring pain. As a physician, I have a responsibility to give hope but also to help the patient prepare for this final phase of life. One gives hope by stressing what medical care can offer with treatment including our ability to control pain. Patients and their family also need to be prepared for what to expect as the tumor progresses and how issues can be addressed. The important message to be conveyed is that the doctor will not abandon them.

Preparing for a productive and meaningful last phase of life isn't easy. Some people live their lives dreading death and they are the living dead. Others continue to be involved and die living. My recommendation to all my patients with advanced disease is to live as though they have two weeks left and during that time make an effort to take care of all their important papers and directives. They then can move on to the next two weeks and hopefully, a few years later will have had a productive and fulfilling life.

I recently came across an article by Dr. Clare Vaughan, a General Practioner in London who wrote about dying from breast cancer in the British Medical Journal (BMJ, V 313, 31 August, 1996, p 565). Her cancer returned after four years of remission, when her youngest child was five years old. She had chemo and was depressed and withdrawn. After a couple of courses of chemo she decided to stop treatments. She wrote that "My heart told me to nurture all the wonderful bits of my life rather than to try and, I suspect unsuccessfully, to poison the tumor." She learned the joy of receiving gifts from friends and loved ones. She also wrote that "In our society people get 'medicalised' and pitied and feared and isolated when they are dying. They have so much to offer if we can just accept it as a time of specialness and privilege. One friend commented that what we really need are midwives for dying."

Sometimes living well and happy is the best palliative medicine I could prescribe. A seventy year old man who had widespread metastatic cancer in the liver and lung came to the office for his routine check-up. He shared that his niece was getting married in California and his entire family was going out there for the event. He really wanted to go but decided against it because of his condition. He was pain free and able to walk and care for himself. I encouraged him to go since he would be surrounded by family and extended family. I told him that if he paced himself and got sufficient rest he should do very well. He made the trip and had a wonderful time, returning home imbued with confidence, living more actively and finally dying a few months later.

Over the years, I have encouraged my patients to use the power of their diagnosis. I would tell them; if there is a loved one or friend from away, invite them to visit. The usual response is that they wish they could get away but can't. However, if told of your condition and that it is not known how long you have, then your request becomes a command performance. This is especially effective during the major holidays such as Christmas or Thanksgiving when adult children are torn between the in-laws and you. I quickly add that if you try that for a couple of years, then you would probably lose your credibility. It upsets me that people drop everything to attend a funeral but don't make the time to visit a failing friend or relative. I suggest to my patients that they tell those close to them that if they make the trip to visit, you will give them a pass from returning for your funeral.

One of the toughest questions I am asked regarding end of life comes from adult children who do not live locally. They very much want to come and spend time with their dying parent but work or young children at home often make it difficult for them to visit for more than a couple of weeks. They often ask me how soon they should come. If the parent fails quickly then the son or daughter would miss out on a final visit. On the other hand, many patients at the end of life rally when out of town children visit since they are stimulated and eat better. I usually encouraged them to come soon-er rather than later.

When I think back over my career, it amazes me how a physician in a white coat can assist a frustrated family and successfully council a patient. Two cases come to mind. One was an eighty year old man who was dying of prostate cancer. His son told me that his father refused to downsize from the large house that his parents lived in for many years and asked me to talk to his dad. I spoke to the patient and he said that he wanted to die in his old house and didn't have the energy or ambition to break it up in his current condition. I pointed out to him that if he did not move, then his elderly wife and children would have to do it after he was gone since she wouldn't be able to live there by herself. He agreed and over the next six weeks they sold their home and moved into a condo in a senior citizen community. On his next visit he was very appreciative of my advice and felt good that he was able to relocate his wife to a safer setting.

Another favorite example of assisting the family with end-of-life decisions involved Sophie, a beloved member of the local Jewish community who was dying of cancer. I went up to one of the floors at Maine Med and I saw her two daughters-in-law leaning against the wall looking distraught. When I asked Joan and Geri what was wrong they told me that their mother-in-law needed to be placed in a nursing facility for end of life care and she refused to consider going to the Cedars Nursing Facility. Cedars had just been built and replaced the old Jewish Home on Munjoy Hill. It was state of the art and considered to be the best in Maine. I offered to speak to her and they encouraged me to do so. I went into her room, gave her a hug and I told her that I heard she did not want to go to the Cedars Facility. She said that the Jewish Home was the place people in our community went to die and she did not want to go there. I reminded her that the Jewish community raised hundreds of thousands of dollars to build the best facility for our community and for the people of Maine. If she and the people we built it for were not going to use it then her message is that we wasted our money. She reluctantly agreed. When I told her daughters-in-law they asked how I did it. I told them it was the power of the white coat. Sophie stayed at Cedars for the remainder of her life and was treated like a queen with many visits from friends and family.

Children, no matter what their age, often play an integral part in their parent's end of life. Whether that is a positive or negative experience only the parent and child can determine, but sometimes a physician can help clear the communication fog and reshape the experience. A patient of mine, a gentleman in his seventies was dying of lung cancer. He told me that he wished his son would stop smoking but he wouldn't listen to him. I asked him if he wanted me to try and he said he would appreciate it. His son was devoted to his dad and brought him in for treatments on most days. I called him in from the waiting room and in front of his dad I told him that his dad asked me to talk to him. I told him if his father could take away the last thirty years of his smoking he would, but he cannot. However, if his illness could be the reason for his son to stop smoking, then his dying of cancer would not be in vain and some good would come of it. Since it was November I told the son that this will probably be his father's last Christmas and the present he would most want would be for him to stop smoking. It would be the least expensive gift he ever gave but one of the most appreciated. I added that his dad knew how difficult stopping smoking would be, but a parent's love is shown by how he protects his child. His son did stop smoking and his father passed away a couple of months later. This is 'hard ball' and puts the child in a very uncomfortable position, but for me, the only time I have to apologize is when I do not take the time to try

A moving end of life story was told to me by a good friend in the local Jewish community. Ellie's elderly parents relocated to an assisted living facility here in Maine to be closer to her. Her dad, who was eighty-six years old had Parkinson's and was becoming more and more frail. Each hospitalization left him weaker and more tired than the one previous. He was failing and he knew it. After yet another hospitalization, he stopped eating. The family knew he had decided it was time to die and they were comfortable respecting his wishes. Six days before his grandson's wedding he lost consciousness at home. Ellie found him and called an ambulance and he was admitted to the hospital for hydration. After twenty-four hours of IV fluids, his daughter was looking out his hospital window and she heard her father's raspy voice saying "What am I doing here?" She knew he meant being alive and in a hospital. She was upset that she wronged him by interfering so she explained that his grandson was getting married that weekend and if he died, her sister and she would not be able to join in the festivities after the ceremony. According to the Jewish religion, if a member of the immediate family passes away, one should not attend a celebration or party during the mourning period that follows. She asked him if he was angry at her and he responded in a soft and gentle voice, "No, I'm not angry". Over the next few days he improved and ate pretty well. Her sister spoke to him by phone shortly after the wedding ceremony on Sunday evening and he passed away the next morning. He had a purpose to live to give his loving daughters and his grandson a final gift so that they could fully participate in this joyful occasion.

The topic of euthanasia, ending life prematurely, came up frequently. I welcomed this discussion and could usually turn it around by emphasizing what the patient can do and how his physicians can keep him comfortable. I also would ask the patient what he would like to do with his remaining time. I reminded him that he will be dead for a long, long, long time. I was unable however to have that conversation with the following young woman since we could not adequately control her symptoms and progression of her disease. She was in her late twenties with a tumor of her palate that was excised but then recurred. It had perineural spread, which is the small space around the nerve routes. She was given chemotherapy and irradiation to the area of the primary and to the draining nerves up to the base of the skull. The tumor returned a couple of years later, was re-resected and recurred again. Other attempts were made to treat her but to no avail. She developed pain and difficulty in maintaining her nutrition in spite of extensive palliative attempts. In her early thirties she decided to give up her fight and had herself admitted to the hospital. I had a long talk with her at which time she said that she could not live like this and that she did not want to die at home in front of her two young daughters. She refused all food and drink in the hospital. She slowly became weaker but because of her young age, she lasted almost four weeks. It was excruciating to watch her fail and it was the only time in my career that I would have considered a physician assisted euthanasia option.

Positive Effects of Cancer Treatment

Several of my patients have told me that sometimes it takes a good swift kick in the butt to appreciate what they have and to no longer sweat the small stuff.

It is difficult to imagine that good can come from a devastating experience such as going through cancer treatment. Many no longer take things for granted and they and their family appreciate one another more. Children of patients when informed of their parent's condition often become helpful and demand less from him or her. The fear of losing that parent will also remind the child how much they need and love that person.

I encourage my patients to accept offers of help and support from friends and neighbors even though this is often difficult for many people. The reality is that friends and family would like to do something to show that they care. They often bake cookies, send flowers or take a half a day to draft a note. I suggest to the patient that they give their friends and family an opportunity to drive them to a treatment every once in a while. By doing this, the well-wisher is contributing in a way that is meaningful and helpful. In addition it is important to give family from out of state an opportunity to come to be of help when a loved one needs it. When a patient tells me that she doesn't want to bother her child, I tell her two things. The first is that the child never worried about bothering her when they needed to be fed or changed. The second was that twenty years from now, that child would like to remember that they spent time with her, during her illness.

The end result, hopefully, is that the patient is cured and that twenty-five years from now, the patient can say that because of their experience with cancer, they appreciated life and their loved ones so much more, and they came to realize that they were loved in a variety of ways by a whole community of friends and family.

ACKNOWLEDGMENTS

This book evolved as a result of my relating to friends and family some meaningful experiences I had with my patients. Carol suggested that I record them before they were forgotten. We agreed that these vignettes would be a good basis for a book that would inform our grandchildren about my professional life. I wrote as if I was dictating a note in a patient's chart with short, boring sentences filled with medical jargon. Carol re-wrote my notes into readable English. Then Moira Lachance used her writing and editing skills to provide invaluable modifications for which I am very grateful.

As I learned over the past couple of years, completing a book is a complex project with contributions from many people. Let me start off with thanking my patients and their families for sharing their cancer experiences with me. I am especially grateful to those patients and family members who reviewed their vignettes, made suggestions and encouraged me to publish their stories.

Providing quality and compassionate medical care is a team effort and I have been very fortunate to work with an outstanding group of individuals throughout my career. The other radiation oncologists, radiotherapists, nurses, dosimetrists, physicists and clerical personnel were a pleasure to work with and I was proud to be associated with them. The Medical staff and administration of Maine Medical Center and our regional hospitals were focused on providing the medical care that we could all be proud of.

Several friends reviewed chapters and made very helpful suggestions. Thank you to Susan Dozier, Joan Levy and to Rabbi Alice Goldfinger for their insightful contributions and to Jim Baker for his Photoshop expertise. Last but certainly not least, I am grateful to Carol's cousin, Barbara Brecher whose professional expertise was indispensable in designing the book cover, formatting the text and shepherding the manuscript into a final product.

Made in the USA
Charleston, SC
25 June 2016